Basic Concepts of EKG

A Simplified Approach

2nd Edition

Harilal Nair
DNP APRN-BC, ANP-C, CCRN, CMC, CSC

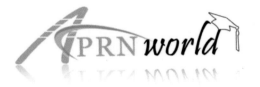

APRN WORLD LLC
California, USA

Disclaimer

This book is designed for both beginners and professionals alike, who are trying to develop better understanding of basic concept of EKG. This book is not a substitution to solid clinical judgment and established medical guidelines for actual patient care. The author and reviewers made tremendous efforts to include most accurate and up to date information in this book. Because of the dynamic nature of modern medicine, the publishers strongly encourage Individual learners to identify most updated information from established and reliable sources for day to day patient care.

ISBN-13: 978-1-941004-10-4

Library of Congress Control Number-2018905250

Publisher Information

APRNWORLD LLC

A digital version of this book is available.

For more info please visit www.aprnworld.com

Preface

Basic concepts of EKG- *A Simplified Approach* **2ⁿᵈ Edition** is an attempt to make the complex nature of EKG analysis to simple and logical endeavor. This edition of the book evolved from the encouragement and feedback that we received for our earlier edition. A 'rationalized approach with simplified analogy' method is again used throughout this book. We strongly believe in the simple to complex and concrete to abstract nature of student learning and therefore, made a substantial effort to deconstruct complex concepts of EKG in to simple building blocks. We would like our readers to consider this book as one of the basic textbooks they use to build a strong foundation for advanced learning.

Every aspect of this book is important in building a stable foundation for further advancement in EKG analysis. Being a constant leaner myself, I don't appreciate books with complex concepts without sufficient explanations. We did our best effort to provide detailed and rational explanations of events whenever possible.

To facilitate multisensory learning of core ideas, appropriate drawings and highlights of important points are included throughout this book. This will enable the students to easily skim through the chapters after initial thorough reading. Important points are color coded and highlighted so that they are more visible than simple detailed mono color paragraphs of the traditional books.

We highly appreciate your comments and looking forward for every opportunity to improve our future products. On behalf of APRN WORLD, I would like to thank my mentors and support team for constant encouragement, support and confidence that they impart on me to make this book a reality.

Sincerely

Harilal Nair DNP APRN-BC, ANP-C, CCRN, CMC, CSC

Thank god

.

Table of Contents

PART 1

BASIC CARDIAC PHYSIOLOGY

Fundamentals of Cardiac Function

In this chapter

- Anatomical location of heart
- Systemic and pulmonary circulation
- Chambers of the heart
- Layers of heart wall
- Micro structure of cardiac cell
- Cardiac cycle
- Coronary circulation
- Nervous system control of heart
- Properties of cardiac cell

Clinical
scenario

Samantha is a student nurse, doing her clinical rotation in the intensive care. She is with Kimberly who is one of the senior nurses in the critical care unit. At change of shift, the night shift RN is giving report on Mr. Robertson who is admitted with congestive heart failure exacerbation. The night shift RN stated 'Mr. Robinson was very sick last night when he came from emergency room. He was bradycardic, hypotensive and having pulmonary edema. Intensivist had to put in a Swan-Ganz and started him on dopamine and furosemide drip. He diuresed overnight and currently much better. This cardiac index and blood pressure improved with the dopamine. But he developed few PVCs in the early morning hours, so please keep an eye on him. I talked to the intensivist this morning and are planning to continue same treatment for now.'. After shift endorsement, Samantha went with Kimberly to meet Mr. Robertson. He was in bed with head of the bed elevated to 45° and on a nasal cannula. When asked by Kimberly, Robertson expressed improvement in his symptoms. He stated 'I was drowning yesterday when I came in, but now feels much better. The night nurse told me I am peeing a lot'. Kimberly said "that's okay Mr. Robertson. With the medications that you are on now, we can get all the extra fluid out of your body without making your heart to work much harder. This will help you to feel better." After initial bedside rounds, Samantha and Kimberly went back to do their routines. Kimberly asked Samantha whether she understood what is happening with Mr. Robertson and why he is on dopamine and Lasix. Samantha replied "I know Lasix is a diuretic that helps to drain extra fluid from Mr. Robertson's body and helps his heart to function well. But I don't quite get the function of dopamine other than it improved his cardiac function. If you don't mind, can you please explain to me that?" Kimberly said " okay, in order to explain things well, let's review the basic anatomy and physiology of our circulatory system".

The heart is a delicate muscular structure lies in the mediastinum and is protected by the rib cage. It is usually situated left of the midline and above the diaphragm. The part of the chest wall overlying mediastinum is called precordium. The apex of the heart is the conical part lies at the bottom and is more towards anterior wall of the chest. Base of the heart is the wider surface along with greater vessels situated on the top. Anatomical variations in position of the heart and greater vessels can be found in cases like *dextrocardia*, where the apex of the heart is rotated towards right side.

pumping blood to the systemic and pulmonary circulations, these chambers have unique role in maintaining various hemodynamic parameters. Therefore, assessment of blood volume, pressure, temperature etc. at various parts of the circulatory system can help in identifying pathophysiologic changes of the heart and other associated structures.

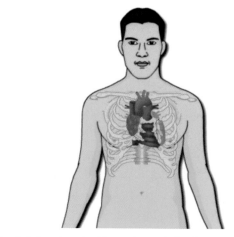

Fig 1.1 Anatomical location of the heart

Circulatory System

The human heart has four pumping chambers known as **right atrium**, **right ventricle**, **left atrium** and **left ventricle**. Along with

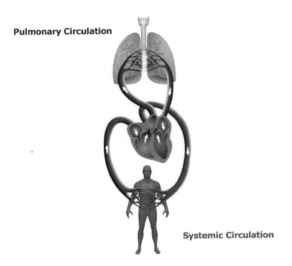

Fig 1.2 Systemic and venous circulation

The heart is a combination of two distinct pumping systems: right pump and left pump. *Right atria and ventricle act as the pump for pulmonary circulation* whereas; *left atria and ventricle constitute the one for systemic circulation*. These two systems are seamlessly connected through the lungs. Both functional units have their own reservoirs (right and left atrium), individual pumping chambers (right and left ventricle) and distinct valve structures that ensure unidirectional flow of blood in the system.

> Absence of flow regulators in the form of valves within the pulmonary circulation helps to balance pressure difference between right and left pumping systems. Left side of the heart has much higher pressure than its counterpart.

Chambers of the Heart

Right atrium This is the *right uppermost chamber* of the heart. The venous circulation from rest of the body empties into the right atrium through *superior and inferior vena cava*. Venous blood from coronary circulation also empties into the right atrium through *coronary sinus*. This chamber has embedded natural pacemaker called *"Sino Atrial node" (SA node)* situated on the right upper corner near the anastomosis of superior and inferior vena cava. Superior and inferior vena cava are the inlet of this chamber whereas, the outlet is one of the atrioventricular valve called *"tricuspid valve"*. It opens towards right ventricle and allows blood flow only in downward direction. The right and left atria are divided by intra-atrial septum.

Right ventricle *Origin of pulmonary circulation* is the significant function of the right ventricle. Blood enters the right ventricle from the right atria through tricuspid valve and exit to pulmonary circulation through *main pulmonary artery*; which later divides into right and left pulmonary trunk. Failure of pumping from the right ventricle results in backing up of venous circulation and clinically manifested by *jugular vein distension* and signs of portal hypertension including

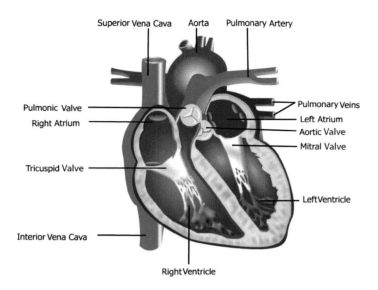

Fig 1.3 Chambers of the heart

peripheral edema. Back flow of blood in to the right ventricle from pulmonary artery is controlled by semilunar valve called *pulmonic valve*.

Left atrium The left atrium receives oxygenated blood from the pulmonary circulation through two pairs of *pulmonary veins*. This oxygenated blood will then pumped into the left ventricle through bicuspid valve called "*mitral valve*". Increased blood volume and pressure within this chamber leads to stagnation of pulmonary circulation, which in turn develop pulmonary congestion.

Left ventricle It is the *most important pumping chamber* of the heart. Majority of cardiac musculature is concentrated here in order to assist in pumping blood against the high-pressure of systemic circulation. Blood from the left atrium comes to the left ventricle through *mitral valve* and exit through *aorta*. The *Aortic valve* situated in between aorta and left ventricle regulates possible back flow of blood during ventricular diastole (relaxation).

Clinical scenario

"okay, now you have seen the heart has four chambers and has two distinct circulatory systems associated with it. But in order to understand the mechanism of heart function, you need to understand bit more about the microscopic structure of the heart. Let's look into that' Kimberly said.

Layers of the Heart Wall

Apart from the three distinct layers of cardiac muscle, the heart is covered in a fibrous double walled sac known as *pericardium*. The surface of the pericardium attached to the chest wall is called *parietal pericardium* and the layer covering the heart is known as *visceral pericardium*. There is a small amount of pericardial fluid between these two layers, which act as a lubricant during the constant movement of heart within the sac. Any excess amount of fluid within this constricted

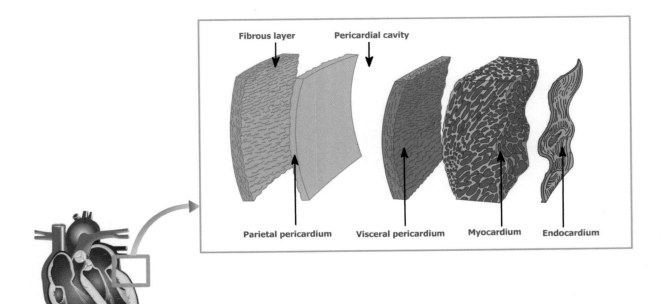

Fig 1.4 Layers of heart wall

space, either in the form of serous fluid or blood effectively obstructs normal pumping function of ventricle and known as *pericardial effusion* and *cardiac tamponade*.

The outermost layer of cardiac muscle is called *epicardium*. The *myocardium* is the middle muscular layer that acts as a mechanism behind pumping function of the heart. Myocardium receives blood supply from the *epicardial coronary arteries* with embedded microvasculature throughout myocardium. The innermost layer called *endocardium* and it covers the inner aspect of all the chambers and other mechanical structures within the heart like heart valves and papillary muscle.

> Up to 1 lit of fluid will not produce any significant symptoms in Pericardial effusion due to the slow rate of accumulation; whereas in cardiac tamponade, 100ml of fluid can compromise hemodynamics because of the fast filling within the pericardium.

Cardiac Muscle Cell

Cardiac myocytes are the building blocks of myocardium, which are striated muscles seen only in the heart. The cross-section of cardiac muscle shows thin and thick protein filaments called *actin and myosin* filaments. These proteins filaments are also known as *myofibrils*. The contracting unit of the myocardium is known as *sarcomere*, which lies between two adjacent dark lines called *Z line* represented by the disk-shaped structure at the end of actin filaments. These fibers are arranged in certain parallel patterns so that, all the fibers will depolarize when any one of them get depolarized.

In the microstructure of actin filament, there are two chains of actin molecules wound about each other on a larger molecule called tropomyosin. A group of regulatory proteins called *troponin C, I* and *T* are spaced in regular intervals on this filament.

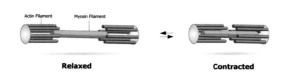

Fig 1.5 Cross-link mechanism

Actin does not have intrinsic enzymatic activity like myosin; however, *in presence of calcium and ATP, actin can reversibly bind with myosin*. In the absence of cellular excitation, tropomyosin prevents cross-linking of actin and myosin filaments. When calcium is present, it combines with the troponin C and forms a confirmatory change for *actin myosin cross-linking*; which in turn causes contraction.

The rate and extent of actin myosin cross bridging continues until the amount of calcium ions fall below a critical level. Therefore, intra cytoplasmic calcium is a principal determinant of myocardial contractility (*ionotropic stimuli*) and is the basis of using various pharmacologic therapies such as cardiac glycosides (e.g. Digoxin), calcium gluconate, calcium channel blockers etc.

> Calcium is the major electrolyte that determines cardiac contractility. In the absence of calcium, myosin and actin cannot form bonds between them and therefore diminishes contraction.

Mechanism of Muscle Contraction

The contracting process of myocardial muscle fibers involve *"sliding filament model"*, where the *thinner actin fibers slide into the thick myosin filaments* during cellular activation. Because of the *tropomyosin*, which is the rod-shaped protein covering all actin myosin binding sites, these filaments are not able to interact each other under normal circumstances.

During cellular activation in response to electrical impulse, *calcium ions* are released into the sarcomere. In the presence of calcium ions, the *troponin*, which is another structural protein that binds tropomyosin to myosin combines with calcium and release tropomyosin bond with myosin receptor sites. This exposes actin and myosin binding sites and promotes both fibers to crawl along each other and facilitate contraction as shown in the picture.

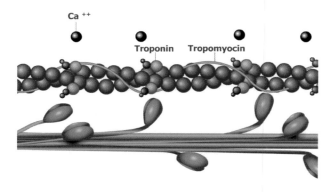

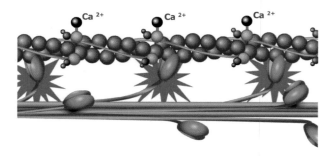

Fig 1.5 (a) Actin and myosin sliding filament action

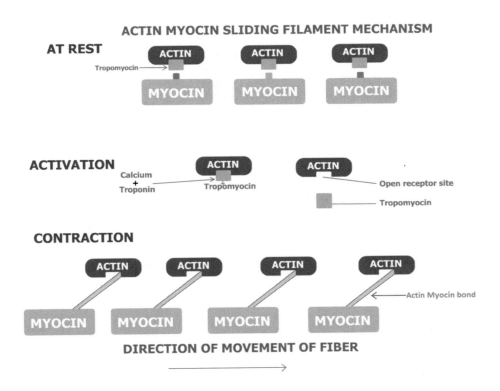

Fig 1.5 (b) Diagrammatic representation of sliding filament theory

In simple terms, consider actin filaments as a spoon and myosin filaments as a can of food. The lid of the can represents tropomyosin, which under normal circumstances prevent the consumer from using the spoon to eat from the can. We have an electric can opener where Troponin is the can opener and calcium ions represent electricity; both together allow us to open the can and access the product. The food will give the consumer energy to work, that is essentially the muscle contraction.

Clinical scenario

"So, is it the same Troponin that is elevated during a heart attack? Samantha asked. "Yes, it is. Troponin is a protein complex seen in skeletal muscles, especially cardiac. During myocardial infarction because of the muscle injury, troponin leaks out of the cell into the blood and can be detected in lab tests. There are three different forms of Troponin seen in skeletal muscles called troponin C, troponin T and troponin I. Among these, troponin I and C are more specific to myocardium and therefore are used as biomarkers of cardiac muscle injury. I'm glad that you're asking all these excellent clinical questions. I hope by the end of the day you will have a better understanding of what is going on with these patients. Now, let's look into what happens during every single beat of the heart. It is very important to know the cycle of events happens with every beat and some new terms like preload and afterload, that explains how the medications work in different clinical scenarios " Kimberly said.

Cardiac Cycle

Cardiac cycle represents the series of events happen with each heartbeat. This process involves systematic filling, open and closure of valves, contraction and expulsion of blood from various chambers etc. Synchronous contraction between heart chambers ensures smooth flow of blood through systemic circulation. Events during cardiac cycle can be broadly divided into *ventricular systole* (contraction), *ventricular diastole* (relaxation), and *atrial systole* (contraction). Fig 1.7 describes various events happen during cardiac cycle.

Determinants of Cardiac Performance

The performance of cardiac muscle depends on three main factors such as the amount of muscle stretch at the beginning of contraction (*preload*), the pressure against which it has to pump (*afterload*) and the force of contraction (*contractility*).

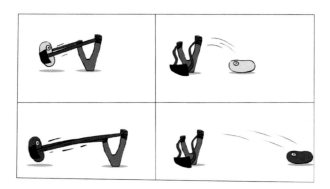

Fig 1.8 A Preload (Frank Sterling's Law; *'The greater the stretch of cardiac muscles, the stronger the contraction'* and resultant force of pumping)

Preload Consider each cardiac muscle as an elastic band. The force of contraction of an elastic band after stretching directly relates to the length of band while it is stretched. The same is true with cardiac muscle. The stretching force of cardiac muscle before contraction corresponds to the volume of blood within the ventricle right before systole [*end diastolic volume/pressure (EDP/EDV)*]. *The higher the volume, stronger the contraction will be*. This relationship is called **Frank Starling's law**. In short, right ventricular preload has a direct relation to the amount of blood coming to the right side of the heart and that is *venous return*.

Afterload: Afterload is the amount of *resistance against which the left ventricle has to pump*. Since left ventricle is pumping blood in to the aorta and systemic circulation, afterload is greatly influenced by systemic vascular resistance (SVR) and BP.

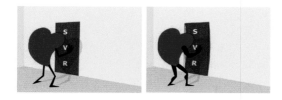

Fig 1.8 B Afterload (Shown as the Systemic Vascular Resistance (SVR) being the force against which the heart pumps blood).

- Preload reducing pharmacologic agents control venous return to the heart mostly by peripheral venous dilatation.

- Afterload reducing agents generally cause peripheral arterial dilation and reduce systemic blood pressure.

- Right ventricle also has afterload, which is determined by pulmonary artery pressure.

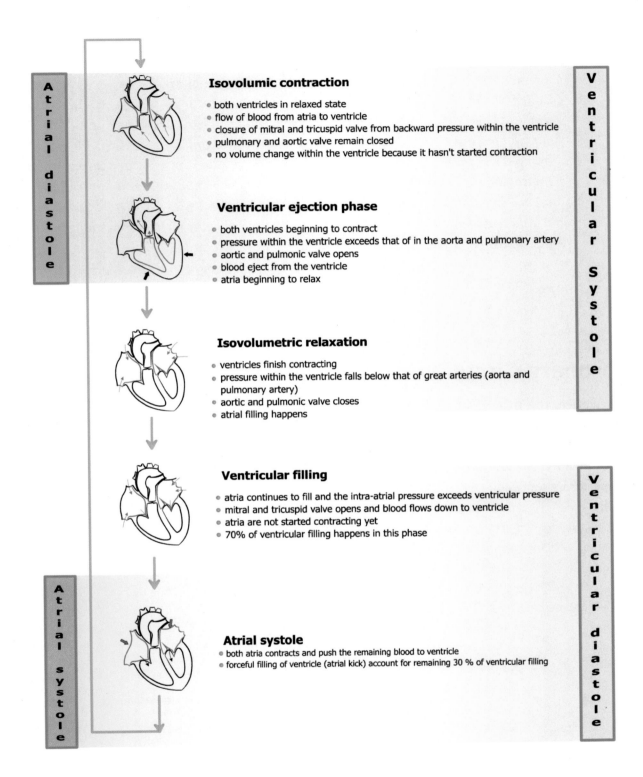

Atrial diastole

Isovolumic contraction

- both ventricles in relaxed state
- flow of blood from atria to ventricle
- closure of mitral and tricuspid valve from backward pressure within the ventricle
- pulmonary and aortic valve remain closed
- no volume change within the ventricle because it hasn't started contraction

Ventricular ejection phase

- both ventricles beginning to contract
- pressure within the ventricle exceeds that of in the aorta and pulmonary artery
- aortic and pulmonic valve opens
- blood eject from the ventricle
- atria beginning to relax

Isovolumetric relaxation

- ventricles finish contracting
- pressure within the ventricle falls below that of great arteries (aorta and pulmonary artery)
- aortic and pulmonic valve closes
- atrial filling happens

Ventricular filling

- atria continues to fill and the intra-atrial pressure exceeds ventricular pressure
- mitral and tricuspid valve opens and blood flows down to ventricle
- atria are not started contracting yet
- 70% of ventricular filling happens in this phase

Atrial systole

- both atria contracts and push the remaining blood to ventricle
- forceful filling of ventricle (atrial kick) account for remaining 30 % of ventricular filling

Ventricular Systole

Ventricular diastole

Fig 1.7   Events during cardiac cycle

After morning routines in ICU, Kimberly and Samantha sat together in front of the computer for charting. Kimberly said," Well, Samantha you have seen the physiology and pumping mechanism of the heart. In the case of Mr. Robertson, dopamine increases the contractility of the of the heart and helps to pump effectively. With a diuretic like Lasix on board, the body then will be able to drain extra fluid out. In simple terms, we can consider the heart as the pump and kidney as the filter. If the pump doesn't pump hard enough, the filter will not filter. By using dopamine, we are improving the contractility of the heart and thereby increasing blood flow in to vital organs like kidney. Now, let's look at how the heart muscles get their blood supply. A concrete idea of coronary circulation is very important for you to understand the mechanism of myocardial infarction and what to look for and where to look for signs of trouble in an EKG. So, listen to this carefully. You may learn more about various aspects of myocardial infarction and their characteristic EKG findings later on."

Coronary Circulation

The heart is the major pumping organ of the body supplying blood to all of the organs. Heart itself gets blood supply through a system of circulation called *coronary circulation*. The coronary arteries supply blood to the myocardium during *diastole*. There are two main coronary artery systems, *Right coronary artery* (RCA)

and *Left main coronary artery* (LMCA). The left main coronary artery supplies two third of the cardiac blood supply. Shortly after its origin from the aorta near aortic cusp, left main coronary artery divides into the *Left anterior descending artery* (LAD) and *Left circumflex artery* (LCx).

Left anterior descending artery (LAD): Left Anterior descending artery

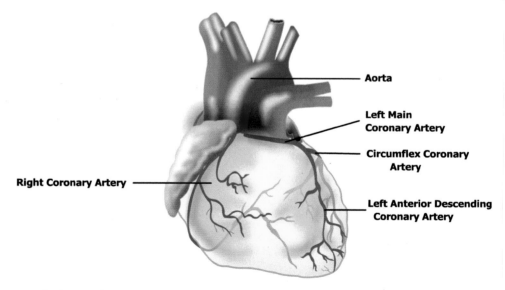

Fig 1.9 Coronary arteries

mainly supplies the *anterior wall of left ventricular myocardium*. It has smaller branches called *Septal perforators* and main branches known as *Diagonal arteries*. LAD has vital role in blood supply to left ventricle. Any occlusion of left anterior descending artery directly affects the pumping function of left ventricle.

Left circumflex artery (LCx): Left circumflex supplies the *lateral and sometimes parts of posterior wall* of the heart. Left circumflex artery give rise to *obtuse marginal branches*.

Right coronary artery (RCA): Right coronary artery feeds the *right ventricle and inferior wall of left ventricle*. Tiny branches of right coronary artery also supply *SA node and AV node*.

> Right coronary artery has a direct effect on heart rate in terms of natural pacemaking function. This is the reason why patients with right coronary artery occlusion and resulting inferior wall myocardial infarction may have bradycardia or various degree of heart block.

Clinical scenario

Around 3 O' clock in the afternoon, Mr. Robertson started having some irregular heart rhythms. He remained in sinus rhythm, but the rates were increasing and decreasing periodically. Kimberly and Samantha went into Mr. Robertson's room. The patient appeared to be sleeping comfortably. Kimberly touched Mr. Roberson's hand and then he woke up. She asked Mr. Robertson how he is doing. Robertson stated "I'm feeling much better. As a matter of fact, I am catching some sleep after last 36 hours. It is always good to sleep without having to wake up feeling like someone is strangling me. I'm fine, thanks for asking". Kimberly replied "you're welcome. Sorry to wake you up, I just wanted to make sure you're okay since there were minor changes in your heart rhythm while you're sleeping". After coming back into the nursing station, Samantha asked "Kimberly, would you please explain what happened and why that happened to Mr Robertson". Kimberly said "you have seen the waxing and waning of heart rate while the patient was sleeping, right? It is sinus arrhythmia. This particular rhythm happens because of the unique nature of nervous system control of the heart. Let's talk little bit about the mechanism of heart rate control".

Nervous System Control of the Heart Rate

The heart is mainly controlled by *autonomic nervous system*. Both divisions of autonomic nervous system such as sympathetic and parasympathetic have effect on heart rate. However, *parasympathetic tone dominates* in healthy young individuals.

> Sympathetic system **increases** automaticity whereas parasympathetic system **inhibits**!!!

In humans, parasympathetic nervous system control is mainly through **vagus nerve**. This

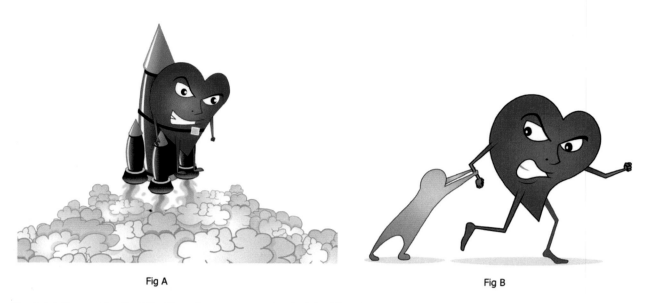

Fig A   Fig B

Fig 1.10 Sympathetic (Fig A) and parasympathetic (Fig B) actions on the heart

nerve originates from the Medulla Oblongata and travel down through the neck near carotid sinus and end at vagal ganglionic cells located around SA and AV nodes. Stimulations of vagal nerve either by *carotid sinus massage* or *Valsalva maneuver* increases parasympathetic influence on SA node and thereby *reduces heart rate*. **Acetylcholine** is the major parasympathetic neurotransmitter for the heart. SA and AV nodes are rich in an enzyme called **cholinesterase** that aids in rapid degradation of acetylcholine. This natural mechanism ensures a rapid decay of any vagal stimulation in the heart.

Rapid beat-to-beat control of heart by vagal response is clinically manifested in patients with *sinus arrhythmia*. In these patients they remain in sinus rhythm during entire sleep, heart rate varies with inspiration and expiration. During expiration, because of the natural vagal stimulation, the heart rate slows down. Even though there is norepinephrine release as part of sympathetic stimulations during inspiration, it does not provide immediate effect on heart rate as the acetylcholine.

Sympathetic innervations of heart originate from lower cervical and higher thoracic part of spinal column. The chemical mediator for sympathetic response is **Norepinephrine**, which has a *slower onset and relatively slow degradation* compared to that of acetylcholine. Therefore, sympathetic stimulation of the heart does not provide a beat-to-beat control as in parasympathetic stimulation. However, the effect lasts longer since Norepinephrine has to be washed away by bloodstream.

Other forms of nervous system control on the heart come from various chemical and pressure receptors. For example, *baroreceptors* located in the aortic arch and carotid sinus mediates a reduction in heart rate when activated. Peripheral chemoreceptors when activated can have vagal response on cardiac activity. A distinct set of sensory receptors located on the endocardial surface of the ventricles are thought to be involved in vasovagal syncope. These receptors are stimulated by reduced ventricular filling volume coupled with vigorous ventricular contraction.

For example, in a person who is standing from a sitting position will have a sudden change in blood volume coming to the ventricle because of the gravitational pooling in abdomen and lower extremities. This leads to a reduction in cardiac output and enhanced sympathetic response. This sympathetic response increases ventricular contraction, which stimulate ventricular receptors leading to profound vagal mediated bradycardia and peripheral arterial vasodilation.

Clinical scenario

At the end of the day, Mr. Robertson appears to be clinically better and was seen by rounding physician who recommended him to be off of dopamine and Lasix drip. He also recommended Mr. Robertson to be transferred to telemetry floor after six hours, provided the patient remains stable. Samantha thanked Kimberly for an excellent clinical day with a lot of exciting knowledge and hands-on experience on a critically ill patient. Samantha also thanked Mr. Robertson for allowing her to take care of him and learned from his clinical scenario. Mr. Robertson expressed his gratefulness to both of them because after all, he is feeling much better and can rest after two days of constant struggle. Kimberly and Samantha wished great evening to each other to be joined on another occasion with a different set of challenges.

Points to Remember!!!

- Four pumping chambers of the heart along with valves perform systemic and pulmonary circulation.
- Systematic and rhythmic contraction and relaxation of these chambers maintain hemodynamics.
- Epicardium, myocardium and endocardium are the three layers of heart wall.
- Within mediastinum, heart is covered with fibrous layer called pericardium with visceral layer attached to heart wall and parietal layer to the inner aspect of chest wall.
- Cardiac contraction is materialized by cardiac myofibrils known as Actin and Myosin filaments.
- Calcium is the major electrolyte determinant of cardiac contraction.
- Cardiac performance is determined by preload, afterload and cardiac contractility.
- Preload is the volume of blood within ventricle right before systole (contraction) and is also known as End diastolic volume (EDV).
- Frank Sterling's law states 'greater the stretch of cardiac muscles before contraction, stronger the contraction will be'.
- Afterload is the amount of resistance against which the ventricle has to pump.
- Three main coronary arteries are Right coronary artery (RCA), Left anterior descending artery (LAD) and left circumflex artery (LCx).
- LAD supplies anterior wall of left ventricle and part of inter ventricular septum

through diagonal branches and septal perforators.

- LCx artery supplies lateral and sometimes part of posterior wall of the heart.
- Right coronary artery supplies inferior wall of heart and mainly structures like SA node and right ventricle.
- Parasympathetic nervous system has more effect on heart rate.
- Parasympathetic system through neurotransmitter called acetylcholine reduces heart rate.
- Vagal nerve is the major parasympathetic control system of the heart.
- Sympathetic nervous system has relatively slow effect through Norepinephrine to the heart compared to that of acetylcholine and is the reason behind sinus arrhythmia.

Test Your Understanding

1. Which of the following represent the inflow valve between right atria atrium and ventricle?
A   Semilunar valves
B   Tricuspid valve
C   Mitral valve
D   Aortic valve   *B*

2. Which of the following structure is not part of pulmonary circulation?
A   Inferior vena cava   *A*
B   Pulmonary Artery
C   Right pulmonary vein
D   Left lung

3. Venous return of myocardial tissue involve_____?
A   Superior vena cava   *C*

B   Pulmonary artery
C   Coronary sinus
D   Pulmonary vein

4. Which of the following clinical symptom is the hallmark of right ventricular failure?
A   Palpitation
B   Jugular vein distention   *B*
C   Dizziness
D   Right-sided chest pain

5. The layer of pericardium attached to the chest wall is called_____?
A   Visceral pericardium *epicardium*
B   Parietal pericardium   *B*
C   Endocardium
D   Myofibrils

6. Which of the following represent the most critical electrolyte in contractility of myocardial cells?
A   Sodium   *C*
B   Magnesium.
C   Calcium
D   Phosphorous

7. Majority of ventricular filling happens during_____?
A   Isovolumetric contraction phase
B   Ventricular filling phase *step1*   *B*
C   Ventricular ejection phase
D   Atrial systole *step 2*

8. Which of the following event during cardiac cycle corresponds to 'atrial kick'?
A   Atrial systole
B   Isovolumic relaxation phase   *A*
C   Ventricular ejection phase
D   Ventricular filling phase

9.Which of the following is true regarding Franks Sterling's law?   A

A   The longer the stretch of cardiac muscle before contraction, the stronger the contraction will be

B   The longer the stretch of muscles before contraction, the weaker the contraction will be

C   The shorter the length of muscles before contraction, the stronger the contraction

D   Contractions are not at all related to the length of muscle stretch

10. Which of the following coronary artery supplies lateral wall of the heart?

A   Posterior descending artery   B

B   Left circumflex artery

C   Septal perforators

D   Right coronary artery   page 11

11. The neurotransmitter believed to have the highest effect on the heart is ___?

A   Norepinephrine

B   Acetylcholine

C   GABA

D   Dopamine

B Vagus nerve controls the S.A node to keep heart rate normal

12. Which of the following neurologic system has most influence on the heart?

A   Sympathetic nervous system   B

B   Parasympathetic nervous system

C   Autonomic nervous system

D   Central nervous system

13. Which of the following accurately represent function of sympathetic nervous system?

A   Slows things down   B

B   Flight fight response

C   Vagal response on the heart

D   Cause peripheral vasodilation

14. Sinus arrhythmia originates from_____?

A   Parasympathetic nervous system

B   Renin Angiotensin system

C   Tropomyosin Calcium complex   A

D   Beta 1 adrenergic receptors

15. Which of the following represent the definition of 'afterload'?   C

A   It corresponds to the stretch of cardiac muscle at the end of diastole

B   It represents the pressure within the ventricle at the beginning of systole

C   It is the pressure against which heart has to pump

D   It has no relation with peripheral vascular resistance

Answers

1.   B   Tricuspid valve
2.   A   Inferior vena cava
3.   C   Coronary sinus
4.   B   Jugular vein distention
5.   B   Parietal pericardium
6.   C   Calcium
7.   B   Ventricular filling phase
8.   A   Atrial systole
9.   A   The longer the stretch of cardiac muscle before contraction, the stronger the contraction will be.
10.   B   Left circumflex artery
11.   B   Acetylcholine
12.   B   Parasympathetic nervous system
13.   B   Flight fight response
14.   A   Parasympathetic nervous system
15.   C   it is the pressure against which heart has to pump

CHAPTER 2

Physiology of Cardiac Contraction

In this chapter

- Electrical properties of myocardial cells
- Normal electrical circuit of the heart
- Cardiac action potential
- Repolarization and depolarization
- Refractory period

Clinical scenario

Bill is a young and energetic boy who recently graduated from high school and joined as the new CCU unit clerk a month ago. He is not only very enthusiastic and hard-working employee but has aspirations for joining nursing school soon. He likes to ask questions about anything and everything he see and hear in CCU to the experienced nurses and doctors he work with. Everyone likes him because of his outgoing person-ality and hardworking nature. Bill is a great help for everyone in the unit. Today Bill is working on CCU Station I where Joyce, who is one of the most experienced CCU nurse is on duty. As usual, Bill doesn't want to miss an opportunity to 'pick Joyce's brain'. As soon as he finished his rush hour tasks, Bill joined Joyce at her desk. Bill asked, " hey Joyce, do you have few minutes to talk? "What is it this time? Last week, you made me explain the entire endocrine system in half an hour. If you continue to do it, I am going to charge you. Fifty bucks per hour". Joyce said with a smile. Bill replied,' "that's ok. Keep a tab on me. I am not going to give up on you. Listen, have you ever heard this, the heart can continue to beat outside for short time after removing from the body? The other day one of my buddy showed me a video on YouTube. It's amazing stuff. How does that happen? Do you believe that? " It is possible". Joyce said. "It is because of the unique nature of cardiac cells. They are very distinct from any other cells in the body because more or less they are self-regulated. Since you asked this question, let me briefly explain the basics properties of cardiac cells." Joyce continued.

The human heart is designed to perform its mechanical pumping function relentlessly through a combination of complex chemical and electrical pathways. In order to provide an appropriate response to electrical stimuli, myocardial cells process charged particles called *ions*. The movements of ions in and out of the cells essentially produce a difference in electrical potential. Specific channels that respond to various stimuli through active and passive mechanisms control this ionic movement.

Properties of Cardiac Cells

Even though autonomic nervous system has effect on cardiac function, the heart doesn't require nervous control for its basic functions. The major cellular properties that distinguish cardiac cells from other tissues are their *contractility*, *conductivity*, *automaticity* and *rhythmicity*.

Contractility is the property by which *cardiac tissue can contract in response to electrical stimuli*. *Conductivity* is the ability of myocardial cells to *conduct electricity after stimulation*. Automaticity and rhythmicity are the major properties that allow perfused heart to beat even when it is completely removed from the body. *Automaticity* is the *ability to initiate its*

own beats and *rhythmicity* is the *capability of maintaining regularity of such pace making activity*.

The capacity of individual cardiac cells to generate, maintain and respond to electrical stimuli serves as a great backup plan in the case of extreme emergencies such as loss of natural pacemaker function. However, the same applies to inappropriate generation, conduction and response of impulses leading to various types of arrhythmias.

By nature, myocardial cells are biologically programmed to respond to the fastest and strongest stimuli available to them. This explains the response of heart towards faster ectopic beats even though the SA node is still producing impulses at lower rates.

Clinical scenario

"So, you think it is absolutely possible for the heart to beat independently outside the body?" Bill asked. "Yes, it is. But I don't know how long and how effective an unsupported cardiac muscle can work outside it's normal surroundings. Because of the inherent properties of cardiac cells as I explained

earlier, it is theoretically possible to generate electricity within the heart and have the muscle respond to it without any external help". Joyce said while filing some papers to the patient's binder. "Now, when you talk about these cellular properties, how does the electricity generated within the cells travel around the heart? Are there any special cells work as electrical wiring?" Bill asked. "Good question". Joyce replied. " Let me finish this charting and then we will look at the electrical pathways within the heart." Joyce replied by typing in the keyboard.

Conduction System of the Heart

Natural electrical circuit of the heart originates from **SA node** and spreads impulse through the surface of atria and down through pathways to the atrioventricular node. In response to an atrial impulse, the chamber contracts and pumps blood through the atrioventricular valves to the lower ventricles. The impulse travels between right and left atria through *Inter atrial pathway* called **Backmann's bundle**. There are three internodal pathways called anterior, middle (Wenckebach) and posterior (Thorel's) tracts exist between SA and AV nodes.

The impulse that reaches atrioventricular node slows down for a time period before spreading downstream. This **AV nodal delay** ensures a *synchronized pumping between upper and lower chambers* of the heart. From the AV node, impulse travels down through pathway known as **Bundle of his**, that further subdivides to right and left bundle branches. The left bundle branch again subdivides into *anterior* and *posterior* division called **fascicles**. The *right and two subdivisions of left bundle* give rise to complex network of **Purkinje fibers**.

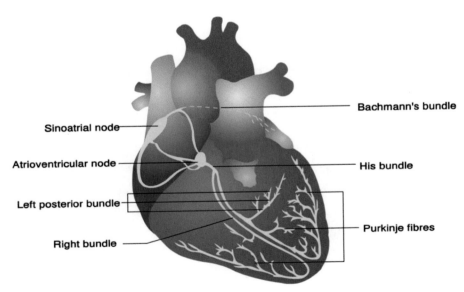

Sinoatrial node

Atrioventricular node

Left posterior bundle

Right bundle

Bachmann's bundle

His bundle

Purkinje fibres

Fig 2.1 Conduction system of the heart

Being the broadest cells within the heart, Purkinje fibers ensures impulse transfer at a higher velocity. This property is key to the immediate activation of entire ventricular myocardium in response to electrical stimuli. These fibers have a long refractory period. It prevents excitation of ventricular tissue in response to inappropriate AV nodal conduction like in the case of atrial fibrillation.

Inherent Rate of Pacemaker Cells

SA node	60 to 100 bpm
AV node	40 to 60 bpm
Ventricle	20 to 40 bpm

The SA node is the natural pacemaker of the heart. In the event of its failure to initiate an impulse, downstream cells start generating electrical impulses in order to maintain cardiac contraction. For example, Junctional rhythm that originates from AV node usually runs at 40 to 60 bpm. If the rate of junctional rhythm is more than 60 bpm, it is called Accelerated junctional rhythm. Similarly, during third-degree heart block or AV dissociation, atrial rate will be somewhere in the order of 60 to 100 beats per minute, whereas ventricular rate usually is in 30 to 40 range.

Box 2.1 Inherent pacemaker rates at various parts of the heart

The myocardial cells in all areas except SA node and AV node polarizes through fast pathway and that ensures rapid conduction of impulse and subsequent repolarization. However, the cells in SA node take calcium mediated slow pathway and are responsible for slow and rhythmic activation of impulses from SA node. These pathways are explained later in this chapter. Various zones within

AV node has *variable conduction velocity* and they help in slowing down impulses (*AV nodal delay*). This process is essential for synchronized electromechanical function of the heart.

In reality, electrical impulse spread through left bundle faster than right bundle. This ensures timely spread of electrical impulses through thick cardiac musculature of left ventricle for synchronized ventricular contraction.

 Clinical scenario

Around noon, one of Joyce's patient developed cardiac arrhythmia while he was sitting in the recliner. Joyce had to call resident physician and subsequently administer electrical cardio version for the patient. Bill was there to help Joyce in getting the patient back in bed at the beginning of the event. Once everything settled, Joyce saw Bill working at a computer terminal and came to thanks him for the help he extended. " You are always welcome. I didn't do anything. You did everything. Even connected him to hundred thousand volts and electrocuted him. Bill replied with a laugh. Joyce padded on his shoulder and said "yeh... I think you may need bit more voltage to get you straight. I will try one of these days..." Okey, let me ask you one thing, Bill said. " Here we go again, Now what?" Joyce asked with a smile. Bill said, "Please explain to me how an erratic rhythm happens like what

happened earlier to your patient, when there is an in-built mechanism of checks and balances between cells at various parts of the heart?". "Well, there are many ways of how things can go wrong. Let me explain a bit." Joyce replied.

Physiology of Cardiac Contraction

As impulses transmitted down through the myocardial cells, they undergo cycles of **depolarization** and **repolarization**. Even though the amount of ionized calcium is the main determinant of cardiac contractility, movement of other ions such as sodium and potassium in and out of the cells are needed to initiate an impulse. The movement of these charged particles create a difference in electrical charge or potential known as

---

Mechanism behind origin of arrhythmia

- Problems with Automaticity (due to suppression or acceleration of phase 4 of cardiac action potential).
  For e.g. sinus bradycardia and sinus tachycardia

- Impaired excitation (suppression of phase 0)
  E.g. Ischemic ventricular fibrillation

- Repolarization issues (premature impulses in phase 3)
  E.g. Polymorphic ventricular tachycardia
  (Torsades de pointes) and atrial fibrillation

Box 2.2 Mechanism behind origin of arrhythmias

---

electrical gradient across the semi permeable cell wall. The *transport of charged particles through active or passive techniques* determines the *nature*, *regularity* and other aspects of myocardial contraction.

There are mainly **five phases** of ionic moments during one contraction process of cardiac cell cycle and is represented by so-called **cardiac action potential curve** as shown in the picture (Fig 2.2). Various phases of cardiac action potential are associated with *changes in permeability of cell membrane to sodium, potassium* and *calcium ions*. There are specific channels for individual ions to go in and out of the cells. The movement of these ions across cell membrane is controlled by factors such as *electrical* and *concentration gradient*.

In the resting state, the cell membrane is relatively permeable to potassium ions compared to sodium and calcium. Therefore, there are *more potassium ions within the cell* compared to surroundings during resting state. However, because of the sheer number of sodium ions present outside the cell compared to the number of potassium ions within, *the interior of the cell has a net negative charge* even though both of these particles are positively charged ions.

Interestingly, the speed of cardiac action potential varies within the heart. There are two types of cardiac action potential known as *fast response* and *slow response* channels. For example, myocytes in *atrial*, ventricular and lower conduction pathways such as *Purkinje fibers* are *fast response type* and therefore can propagate the impulse at *higher speeds* and respond accordingly. At the same time, the cells in *Sino atrial node (S A node) and atrioventricular node (AV node) are slow response* type. This difference in response behavior helps to *control the rate of cardiac activation* at physiologically appropriate levels.

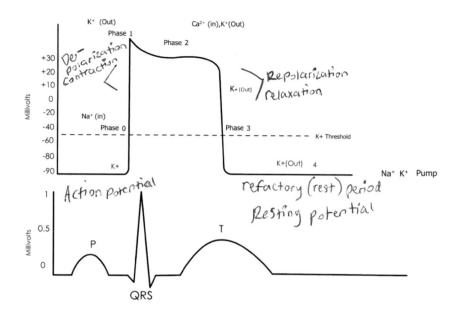

Fig 2.2 Action potential of ventricular myocytes

The innate property of *response time differ-ence* between these two distinct areas ensures the function of SA node as a natural pacemaker. Rhythmic impulses produced by SA node then spread across myocardium at a faster pace. At the AV node, the impulses again slow down and then propagate downstream. This AV nodal delay provides enough time for a sequential contraction of atria followed by ventricles.

Cardiac Action Potential

Cardiac action potential represents the series of ionic moments within myocardial cells and resulting electrical current that trigger muscle contraction. Various myocardial cells have slightly different action potential in the form of slow and fast response pathways as mentioned earlier. For the sake of simplicity, we will analyze action potential of a ventricular cardiomyocyte, which is the common myocardial cell.

The basic principle of action potential is that the cell always tries to come back to its resting electrical state even after disturbance in electrical charge.

Phase 0

Any electrical stimulus that abruptly changes the resting membrane potential to the threshold level generates an *action potential*. At this phase, there is a sudden *influx of sodium ions* into the cell from outside through specific channels called **fast sodium channels**. This accounts for the steep *upslope of phase 0* in the action potential representation curve. Now, because of the large influx of sodium ions that are positively charged, it effectively neutralizes existing negative charge within the cell. Consequently, the interior of the cell becomes more and more positively charged.

Phase 1

This is represented by the area between the *end of upstroke* (*Phase 0*) *and the beginning of plateau* in the action potential representation. During this phase, activation of potassium channels leads to *outward flow of potassium* ions from the cells. This process results in a partial and brief period of repolarization of the cell.

Phase 2

> Slow response cells in the heart such as SA node and AV junction are depolarized not through the fast sodium channels, but through slow calcium channels. The repolarization is achieved by inactivation of calcium channels and increased outflow of potassium during phase 3.

Calcium ions are the main players in this phase of cardiac action potential. In this phase the *calcium ions enters through calcium channels*, which are much *slower than the fast sodium channels*. Simultaneous *outflow of potassium ions* continues from phase 1. This inward and outward movement of positively charged ions effectively counterbalance electrical gradient during this phase.

Phase 3

The process of final repolarization starts when the amount of *potassium outflow exceeds influx of calcium ions*. Outward movement of potassium is highest during this phase and it results in bringing electro negativity within the cell. Towards the end of phase 3, sodium and calcium channels are completely closed.

Phase 4

During this phase, the excess of sodium that got into the cell during initial part of cardiac action potential is eliminated by **active sodium potassium ATPase pump**. This leads to increasing negativity within the cell. During this active sodium elimination process, three *sodium ions are exchanged for two potassium ions* within the cell and hence, more intracellular potassium than sodium as in the resting state. Excess of calcium also expelled through **active calcium pump** during this phase. Altogether, the cell repolarizes back to baseline and another action potential cycle begins. Various ionic movements during cardiac action potential are summarized in the table below.

Major Ionic Movement to Intracellular space in Cardiac Action Potential

Ion	Phase 0	Phase 1	Phase 2	Phase 3	Phase 4
Sodium	Large amount moves in				Three Sodium ions move out*
Potassium		Going Out	Going out	Going out	2 Potassium ions Move in *
Calcium			Going in	Going in	Going out

*Sodium Potassium pump

Table 2.1 Ionic movements in cardiac action potential

Various drugs and sympathetic neurotransmitters such as beta-receptor agonist (Isoproterenol) and norepinephrine enhance calcium in flow. Parasympathetic neurotransmitter such as acetylcholine may reduce calcium conductance. These properties are the basis of using calcium channel blockers like Verapamil and Diltiazem.

Due to the blockade of calcium channels, these agents effectively reduce the duration of phase 2 of cardiac action potential and diminish the strength of cardiac contraction. This in turn depresses vascular muscle contraction and thereby produces generalized vasodilatation. Therefore, these agents are called afterload reductors.

Clinical scenario

John who is a student nurse, was overhearing what Joyce and Bill were discussing about the cardiac action potential. He turned around and asked, "Sorry to interrupt your conversation. Shall I join too?". " No, this is an exclusive club. You cannot interfere". Bill said with a serious expression on his face. He then quickly changed his expression and said "Sorry man, I was joking. You are most welcome to join. This is a brain picking session. Joyce has one of the best you can ever pick. She is awesome. Joyce, do you mind John joining?" Bill asked Joyce. "Absolutely not, I am more than happy to tell you guys what I know". Joyce replied. John asked, "Well, I was always puzzled with the term refractory period. Can you explain to me in simple terms?" "Certainly", Joyce said. She then grabbed a piece of paper from the stack at the corner and start drawing an action potential curve. "Okay, let me explain a bit and then we will look at this picture.".

Refractory Period

Refractory period is a certain timeframe during each cycle of cardiac action potential where the cells are *not capable of* responding to

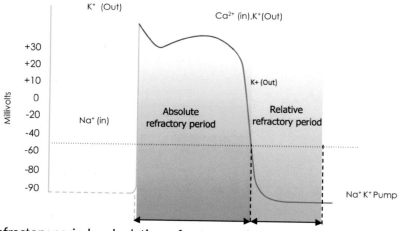

Fig 2.3 Absolute refractory period and relative refractory period

if heart responds here before new cycle = Sinus arrythmia

another electrical stimuli. There are two types of refractory period known as **Absolute** refractory period and **Relative** refractory period.

Absolute refractory period is the interval from the *beginning of phase 0 of action potential to a point in phase 3* at which the depolarization has reached about -50 mV. During the rest of phase 3, a subsequent cardiac action potential *may be provoked if the impulse is strong enough*. Patients with premature electrical beats may have clinical consequences if the impulse originates early in phase 3. During this moment, the conduction of premature impulse from the *site of origin will be slow* and therefore *higher chance of re-entry* that leads to dangerous arrhythmias like **ventricular fibrillation**.

Clinical scenario

At the end of the day, John and bill were very happy to learn few new things about the physiology of cardiac function. Joyce was happy as her patient was saved well before any hemodynamic compromise from a very fast heart rhythm because of her timely intervention. It was a good day in the unit for everyone involved.

Points to Remember!!!

- Major properties of cardiac cells are contractility, conductivity, automaticity and rhythmicity.
- Automaticity is the ability to generate its own impulse and conductivity is the ability to conduct those impulses. Contractility is the property of contraction in response to those impulses and rhythmicity is the ability to maintain rhythmic contractions.
- Myocardial cells have the inherent property to respond to the fastest stimuli available to them.
- SA node, AV node, Bundle of his and Purkinjee fibers grossly constitute the conduction system of the heart.
- Inherent rate of SA node is 60-100 bpm and the rate of impulse production progressively slows down in cells down the line within conduction system.
- Inherent pacemaker rate of junctional tissue is 40-60 bpm and that of ventricle is 20-40 bpm.
- When a rhythm exceeds its inherent impulse production rate, it is called 'accelerated rhythm'.
- Cardiac action potential curve represents the electrochemical events during myocardial activity.
- Movement of sodium in to the cells represents upstroke or phase 0 of cardiac action potential.
- Outward flow of potassium ions constitutes Phase 1.
- Inflow of calcium ions through slow sodium channels corresponds to Phase 2 of action potential curve.
- In phase 3, continuing outward flow of potassium exceeds inflow of calcium.
- In phase 4, active sodium potassium pumps and calcium pumps move ions around, resulting higher concentration of potassium within the cell as in the beginning of phase 0.
- Refractory period is the timeframe within action potential curve where the cell is not capable of responding to another electrical stimuli.

- Absolute refractory period is the time between Phase 0 to a point in Phase 3 where the tissue is incapable of depolarization no matter how strong the impulse is.
- Relative refractory period is the time in which a sufficiently stronger stimulus can produce a premature impulse.

Test Your Understanding

1. Which of the following represent the natural properties of myocardial cell that aids in generation of electrical impulses?
A   Conductivity
B   Contractility
C   Automaticity
D   Refractory period

2. Which of the following statement is true regarding the nature of cardiac cells?
A   Myocardial cells respond to the strongest and fastest stimuli available to them
B   Myocardial cells respond to the weakest and slowest stimuli available to them
C   Myocardial cells do not respond to electrical stimuli other than from SA node
D   Myocardial cells only respond to electrical stimuli from SA node no matter how fast or slow they are

3. Which of the following structure is part of conduction system of the heart?
A   Aortic annulus
B   Atrioventricular node
C   Mitral valve
D   Left atrial appendage

4. Inherent pacemaker rate of ventricular tissue under normal circumstances is _____?
A   150-150 bpm
B   45-60 bpm
C   20-40 bpm
D   P0-100 bpm

5. Which one of the following physiologic mechanism ensures a synchronized atrio ventricular contraction?
A   Phase 0 of action potential
B   AV nodal delay
C   Presence of calcium
D   Slow response channels within SA node

6. Which of the following phase of cardiac action potential corresponds with inward movement of sodium to the cell?
A   Phase 3
B   Phase 1
C   Phase 4
D   Phase 0

7. Which of the following statement is true regarding electrical charge at resting cardiac cell?
A   There are more negatively charged particles outside the cell compared to intracellular fluid
B   There are more positively charged particles inside the cell compared to extracellular fluid
C   There are more potassium ions outside the cell compared to sodium
D   There are more sodium ions outside compared to intracellular potassium

8. The net electrical charge of intracellular fluid is _____?
A   Positive

B   Negative
C   Neutral
D   Unable to determine

9. Which of the following phase of cardiac cycle involves major action of sodium-potassium pump?
A   Phase 1
B   Phase 2
C   Phase 0
D   Phase 4

10. Which of the following statement is true regarding absolute refractory period?
A   Absolute refractory period represent the peak point of QRS complex
B   This is the time when an external impulse can create cardiac action potential
C   This is a time when the cell is incapable of responding to any external stimuli

D   This is the time frame in which heart rest between contractions

Answers

1.   C   Automaticity
2.   A   Myocardial cells respond to the strongest and fastest stimuli available to them
3.   B   Atrioventricular node
4.   C   20-40 bpm
5.   B   AV nodal delay
6.   D   Phase 0
7.   D   There are more sodium ions outside compared to intracellular potassium
8.   B   Negative
9.   D   Phase 4
10.   C   This is a time when the cell is incapable of responding to any external stimuli

CHAPTER 3

Basics of EKG

In this chapter
- Basic concepts of EKG
- Components of EKG wave
- Various lead placements
- Identifying EKG wave forms
- Intervals and measurements
- Unipolar and bipolar leads and its significance

Clinical scenario

Michele is one of the telemetry RN who joined the unit yesterday. She was working in Maternal and child health unit for last twelve years. Since she is new to the unit, Michele is orienting with Barbara, a veteran at the unit. Today on her first day on the job, Michele told Barbara, " Honestly, I am very nervous. After being in OBGYN unit, I completely forgot about the EKG and its technicalities. Unit educator Terry told me you are very good at explaining everything there is to know about EKG and many other things. I hope you don't mind spending some time with me". " Oh, no. It's my pleasure to work with you. I really enjoy people like you who ask question about something that you don't know rather than faking it and later on getting in trouble. I am more than happy to explain to you what I know. But I just want to tell you one thing. I don't know everything. If I don't know something, I will tell you that. But we can ask someone else and find the answer". Barbara said. "Thank you so much for making me comfortable in this unit. Your words are really encouraging for me". Michele replied. "Okay, let me explain to you some of the basics of EKG since we have a little time before we pass morning medications." Barbara replied by reaching to the wall cabinet at nurse's station. She grabbed an EKG manual and started explaining.

The electrocardiogram is a graphical representation of electrical activity of the heart. Devised in the early part of 20th-century, EKG became an integral part of screening, diagnosis and management of cardiac diseases in medicine. Each individual lead in the EKG shows electrical activity between two different parts of the body. This minute electrical activity is measured, magnified and graphically represented in various forms in electrocardiogram. The heart being a three-dimensional structure involving three planes, it needs more than one view to assess activity along all surfaces. This is how EKG with more than one lead has evolved.

Most commonly EKG can be single lead, two leads, three leads, six leads and 12 leads depending on the number of leads in use. In a *12 lead EKG* we're looking at the heart from *12 different views*, six in vertical and other six in horizontal direction. These views provide most comprehensive outlook of electrical activity and is especially helpful in diagnosing events involving a localized area of the heart. A 12 lead EKG provides valuable information regarding anatomical orientation of the heart, chamber size, influence of drugs, some electrolyte imbalance, presence and extent of ischemic changes, abnormal conduction pathways etc. Considering all these benefits, it is impressive to see how much vital health information can be provided through this simple, least expensive and probably most accessible diagnostic exam which hasn't changed much over the last 100 years.

[handwritten: Connection of the ~~right~~ Machine to the body]

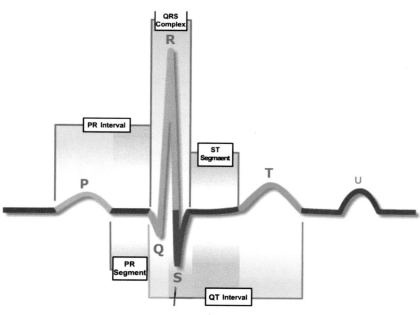

Fig 3.1 **PQRST complex and Intervals**

[handwritten: electrical activity to both ventricles]

In general, the EKG tracing consists of waveforms named P, Q, R, S, T and occasionally U waves. Individual waves represent electrical activity happens in various parts of the heart. *Since the electrical activity is synchronized with mechanical function, EKG tracing indirectly represent contraction and relaxation of various chambers.* Considering the electrical excitation and ion transfer at molecular level, these waves also helps in identifying physical, physiologic and pathologic changes in cardiac cells.

flowing. Whenever the *current flows towards the positive electrode*, we will see an *up stroke* or *positive spike* in the EKG. The reverse happens when current flows toward *negative* electrode. A *biphasic* or *isoelectric* complex generates when the direction of flow is *perpendicular* to the positive electrode.

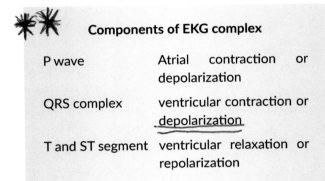

Components of EKG complex

P wave	Atrial contraction or depolarization
QRS complex	ventricular contraction or depolarization
T and ST segment	ventricular relaxation or repolarization

Box 3.1 Components of EKG complex

"But I don't understand why these EKG waves are going all over the places. Some are pointing up, some down and some in between. It is kind of confusing". Michele said. "Hey, Tammy, can you please give me a sheet of scratch paper", Barbara asked Tammy who is the monitor tech at the unit. Tammy handed over a piece of paper to Barbara. She started drawing and said' Okay, Michele, let me explain".

Wave Morphology

The direction of complexes in an EKG is determined by the direction towards the current is

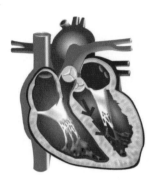

Fig 3.2 Net direction of electrical current in the heart

This is of great help in understanding morphology of various EKG leads. Because of the large muscle mass concentration in the left ventricle, *the net vector (direction) of electricity in the heart is generally directed towards left and downward direction*.

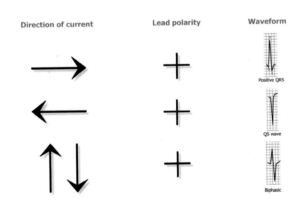

Fig 3.3 Wave morphology and direction of current flow

Therefore, any lead that is closer to the left ventricle such as precordial leads V4, V5 and V6 may see large electrical activity in the form

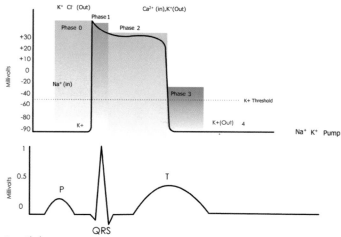

Fig 3.4 EKG and action potential

of **tall R waves**. Similarly, in V1 which is situated on the right sternal border; the direction of flow of current is away from it and therefore predominantly negative in nature. This basic idea applies to all the limbs leads and augmented leads in an EKG.

> **Current flowing** towards positive electrode generate positive **waveform and** away from it generate negative **waveform.**

Clinical scenario

Later in the day, Barbara and Michele got a new admission from ER, Mr. Johnson, a 58-year-old male with chest pain. After an hour in the telemetry unit, Mr. Johnson complained about some heaviness in his chest. While preparing Mr. Johnson for 12 lead EKG, Barbara asked the patient, "Mr. Johnson, how are you feeling after I gave you that nitroglycerin pill under your tongue?" Patient replied "I am actually beginning to feel better. I feel like the heaviness

is going away". She then turned around and explained to Michele, "let me tell you one thing. It's very important to know how to place the lead correctly while taking a 12 lead because it can affect what we can interpret from the tracing. If you don't place it correct, important things can get missed. So, let me explain it to you. Don't worry if you don't get it at the first time. Practice makes it perfect. So, keep doing it by looking at the diagram on the wall", Barbara said while pointing to the Lead placement diagram at the head of the bed.

Lead Placements in a 12 lead EKG

In order to place precordial leads accurately on the chest, we have to follow some anatomical landmarks and imaginary lines on the chest

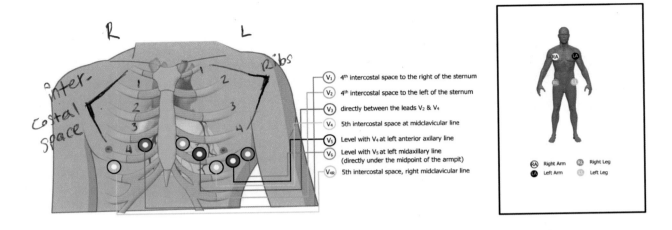

Fig 3.5 **Lead placement in EKG**

wall. Since the intensity of electrical activity from the heart diminishes as the electrode placement moves away, *inaccurate lead placement results in poor and low amplitude EKG tracing.* The locations of individual leads are carefully determined in relation to the area of the heart under scrutiny.

Lead V1 sits close to right ventricle and should be placed on the space between fourth and fifth ribs along the right border of the sternum. Similarly, lead V2 is placed on the same location but on the left sternal border. Usually lead V3 is placed after V4 because the location of V3 is defined as 'in between V2 and V4'.

Lead V4 follows an imaginary line drawn from middle of the left clavicle known as midclavicular line (MCL) and usually falls below the nipple line. V5 follow the imaginary line coming down from the beginning of patient's left armpit known as anterior axillary line (AAL). Lead V6 goes under the left armpit on the imaginary line dividing the axilla known as mid axillary line (MAL).

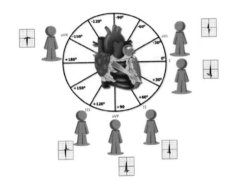

Fig 3.6 **View of the heart from various lead positions**

Posterior structures of the heart such as right atrium, posterior wall etc. are not well visualized in the regular 12 lead EKG setup. Therefore, we can add specific leads looking at the structures either on the right side of the heart or towards the posterior chest wall. Most common leads used for these purposes are lead V3R and V4R. They assume similar positions as its counterparts on the left chest wall. We also can have lead V7, V8 and V9, which are placed on the posterior chest wall similar to that of lead placement on the anterior wall, but as in mirror image.

Location of chest leads

V1	Fourth intercostal space on the right sternal border
V2	Fourth intercostal space on the left sternal border
V3	Between V2 and V4
V4	Fifth intercostal space in the left mid-clavicular line
V5	Fifth intercostal space in the left anterior axillary line
V6	Fifth intercostal space in the left mid-axillary line
V3 R	Between V1 and V4R
V4R	Fifth intercostal space on the *right mid-clavicular* line

Box 3.2 Location of chest lead placement

Clinical scenario

In the afternoon, once Mr. Johnson was seen by the cardiologist and taken to the cardiac cath lab for coronary angiogram, Barbara sits down with Michele to help with her charting. Once the work finished, Michelle asked, " Hey Barbara, earlier I saw you measuring something in the EKG strip of Mr. Chandler in Room 12. What was it about? " Barbara replied, "Oh, I was measuring the QT interval on that patient. Remember, he had Amiodarone due at that time. It is one of those drugs that can prolong the QT interval". "Sorry, can you please explain a bit more" Michelle asked. "Well, let me get a telemetry strip". Barbara got up and walked towards the central monitor and came back with a printed strip. " So, this is the strip for Mr. Chandler. Now before start measuring, let me explain the basics of EKG paper. I will also explain how to identify each wave form in an EKG strip". Barbara said.

Electrocardiography Paper

Traditionally EKG is recorded in a graph paper that is divided into small and large columns. In a running strip, **X axis** (from left-to-right) indicates the *time* and **Y axis** (bottom to top) represents *voltage*. Typically, the speed at which EKG recording happens is 25 mm per second. If the complexes are too narrow and clustered together as in tachyarrhythmia, the speed of EKG recording can be doubled, which helps in widening the waveforms and possibly better identification of the rhythm.

As shown in fig 3.7, each *small box* from *left-to-right* indicates *0.04 seconds*. Since one large box includes five small boxes, *each large box* represents *0.2 seconds (0.04 sec x 5 = 0.2 sec)*. There are five large boxes in one second (0.2 sec x 5 =1.0 sec). Usually there are three second markings on the top or bottom of the EKG paper and it helps in calculating rate of contraction as explained later in this chapter. In the same manner, each *small box* from *bottom to top* indicates *0.1 mV* and therefore, a stack of *10 boxes* in *Y-axis* represents *1 mV (0.1mV x 10= 1.0 mV*. These measurements are critical in determining various intervals and pathologic conditions from an EKG strip.

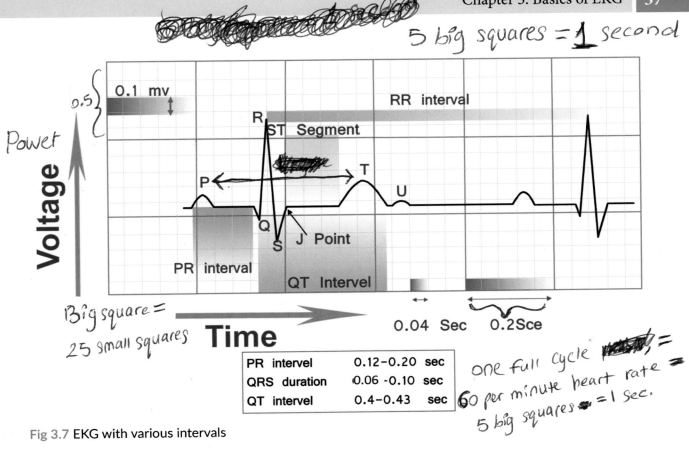

Fig 3.7 EKG with various intervals

PR intervel	0.12–0.20	sec
QRS duration	0.06 -0.10	sec
QT interval	0.4–0.43	sec

Intervals and measurement in EKG

PR interval   *Time delay in conduction of impulse in the AV node.*
It is prolonged in some types of heart block.
Normal 0.12 to 0.20 seconds

QRS duration   *Time of ventricular repolarization (contraction).*
This value is increased in bundle branch block and premature ventricular contraction.
Normal 0.06 to 0.10 seconds.

QT interval   *Total time of cardiac contraction and relaxation.*
Drugs like Amiodarone elongates QT interval.
Normal 0.40 to 0.43 seconds

Box 3.3 Various intervals in EKG

Corrected QT Interval (QTc)

QT interval in an EKG depends on the heart rate. With faster heart rates, QT interval is shorter as there is less time between repolarization and depolarization cycles. Conversely, QT interval is long with slower heart rate. If the given EKG has tachycardia or bradycardia, it can mask an underlying abnormal QT interval. Since the QT interval is extremely important in recognizing potential for lethal arrhythmia, a corrected QT interval (QTc) for a given heart rate should be calculated in every rhythm strip. One of the common QTc calculation formula is called Bazett's Formula and is shown below.

$$QT_c = \frac{QT}{\sqrt{RR}}$$

where

      QTc is the corrected QT interval for the given heart rate

      QT is the measured QT interval from the EKG strip

      RR is the distance between two consecutive R waves (RR interval)

It is important to remember that corrected QT interval is closely connected to heart rate and therefore calculating QTC on irregular rhythms such as Atrial fibrillation is very challenging. One of the common method used for measuring QTC in Atrial fibrillation is that the final corrected QT interval is the average of the QTc of two subsequent long and short QRS complexes as shown below.

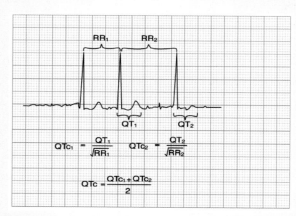

Fig 3.7B Calculating QTC in Afib

Box 3.5 Corrected QT interval

Identification of Waves in EKG

P wave	*First positive deflection* in the EKG complex. It is inverted in the junctional rhythm or in aVR, V1 and in some pathologic waves. It determines whether the impulses are originating from the atria or somewhere else.
Q wave	*First negative deflection* in the QRS complex. A large Q wave (Greater than 0.04 ms and greater than one third of R wave) represents myocardial death.
R wave	*Second positive reflection* in PQRST complex. It is usually tall in EKG leads with a positive electrode on the left side of the chest wall such as lead I, II, III, aVL, aVF, V5 and V6.
S wave	*Second negative deflection* in the PQRST complex.
T wave	*Third positive deflection* in the EKG complex. In ischemia or infarction, T waves may be inverted.
U wave	*4th positive reflection* immediately following the T wave.
J point	*The junction between end of QRS and the beginning of ST segment.* **J** point is elevated in ST Elevation Myocardial infarction (STEMI)

Box 3.4 Waveforms in EKG complex

Clinical scenario

"Well, I have a question about the leads. Earlier I saw the Cardiologist asking the monitor tech to change the monitoring leads on Mr. Johnson while he had chest pain. He told her to change to bipolar leads. I didn't get that." Michelle said. Let's walk to the pharmacy to pick up this antibiotic for Mrs. Sanchez in Bed 14. It's almost time and pharmacy hasn't delivered it yet. Since we don't have any aids today, we have to go and pick it up to be given on time." Barbara said while getting up from her chair. While walking down the hall, Barbara explained.

Various Leads in Electrocardiography

Even though the EKG represents electrical activity of a live organ, for an electrocardiogram machine it is simply the difference in electrical potential between two given points called *leads*. Depending on the number of physical leads needed for this calculation, it can be classified into bipolar (lead I, lead II and lead III) and unipolar leads (aVR, aVL, aVF and all V leads).

Bipolar Leads

These are the basic leads proposed by William Einthoven, who was the Nobel Prize winner in 1924 for invention of practical

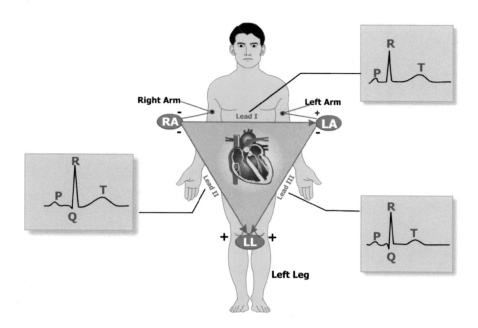

Fig 3.8 Einthoven triangle and limb leads

electrocardiogram. According to him, the *'sum of the heights' of QRS in leads I and III equals the height of QRS in lead II.* This equation is called **Einthoven's law.**

As shown in the picture, lead I has negative electrode on the right arm and positive on the left arm. Since the direction of current in the heart is towards left side and the positive electrode is sitting on the left arm in this case (flow of current towards positive electrode), *lead I* will have a *positive QRS* under normal circumstances. In *lead II*, right arm is negative and left leg is positive and direction of current is again towards positive electrode; resulting EKG will be predominantly *positive*. In lead III, potential difference is measured between the left arm and left leg with a positive electrode as shown in the picture, resulting EKG will be positive. Among these three leads, *lead II* will have *tallest R* waves since lead II closely

represent the *true direction of the net cardiac vector.*

Unipolar Leads

Unlike bipolar leads, unipolar leads have a single physical electrode attached to the body. The machine calculates *electrical difference between the single available lead and an imaginary point at the center of the heart with Zero electrical potential.* Among these, lead **aVR, aVL** and **aVF** are known as **Augmented leads** because the machine has to increase or augment EKG tracing by 50% for the purpose of representation.

All precordial leads like V1 to V6, right-sided precordial leads like V3R, V4R and posterior precordial leads such as V7, V8 etc. are unipolar like augmented limb leads. Posterior leads such as V7, V8 and right-sided precordial leads such as V4R, V5R may be recorded for special circumstances as in posterior wall myocardial infarction. Posterior wall MI results from occlusion of dominant circumflex coronary artery or dominant right coronary with large posterolateral branch. In these conditions, anterior precordial leads may only show '*reciprocal changes*' due to a ST elevation MI. These lead placements are the mirror image of left-sided anterior precordial leads on their corresponding body surface.

> Remember, if there is no QRS complex, there is no cardiac output!!!

Clinical scenario

At the end of the day, Michelle felt like she got a handle on things at her new unit. She felt more comfortable taking care of patients in the telemetry unit. Even though they are entirely different from her old group of maternity patients, she was so happy that she is learning new and interesting things. At last EKG is not that scary to her as it was before. Barbara was happy that Michelle was very receptive to her guidance and felt like she is going to be a great addition to the crew in telemetry unit. Mr. Johnson got angiogram and had a stent placed in left anterior descending artery. He came back to the unit right at the change of shift, so both Michelle and Barbara couldn't get to spend time with him after the procedure. But they were happy that his problem was taken care of.

Points to Remember!!!

- EKG is the graphical representation of the electrical activity of the heart.
- Each individual EKG leads show electrical activity between two different parts of the body.
- In 12 lead EKG, we are looking at six horizontal and six vertical angles at the heart.
- Current flowing towards the positive electrode shows a positive waveform in EKG and that flows away from positive electrode give negative waveform.
- The net vector (direction) of electrical activity of the heart is directed towards left and downward direction (towards left ventricle).
- Leads closer to the area of the heart with the net direction of current show tall positive waveforms (Lead V5, V6).
- Since EKG waves indirectly represent cardiac contraction, 'absence of QRS' means no ventricular contraction and therefore, no cardiac output'.
- Right sided and posterior leads are utilized in assessment of posterior walls of the heart.
- In EKG graph, from left to right (X axis) is the 'time' and from bottom to top (Y axis) is the 'voltage'.
- Each small box in an EKG grid represents 0.04 sec in X-axis and 0.1 mV in Y-axis.
- PR interval is the delay in conduction of impulse from the SA node to AV node (0.12-0.20).
- QRS complex represents time of ventricular contraction (0.06-0.10 sec).
- QT interval is the total duration of ventricular contraction and relaxation (0.40 - 0.43 Sec).

- Lead I, II, III are called bipolar leads and Lead aVR, aVL, aVF and V1-V6 are unipolar leads.

Test Your Understanding

1. Which of the following represent QRS complex in an EKG?
A   Ventricular contraction
B   Ventricular diastole
C   Atrial systole
D   Atrial contraction

2. Which of the following statement is true regarding direction of current and EKG waveform?
A   Current flowing towards negative electrode produces a positive waveform
B   Current flowing away from negative electrode produces a negative waveform
C   Current flowing towards the positive electrode produces a biphasic waveform
D   Current flowing away from positive electrode produces a negative waveform

3. The net direction of electrical activity of the heart is directed towards_____?
A   Right atrial appendage
B   Right ventricular outflow tract
C   Left ventricle
D   Sino atrial node

4. In a normal heart, which of the following represents the direction of EKG complex in lead V6?
A   Isoelectric
B   Positive
C   Negative
D   Varying from person to person

5. Which of the following precordial lead is placed in the fifth intercostal space at anterior axillary line?
A   Lead V2
B   Lead V6
C   Lead V5
D   Lead V3

6. Which of the following parameter is displayed on X axis of EKG?
A   Time
B   Voltage
C   Heart rate
D   Force of contraction

7. Normal QRS complex duration is _____?
A   0.12-0.2 second
B   0.40-0.43 second
C   0.06-0.10 seconds
D   0.24- 0.30 seconds

8. Which one of the following is an example for bipolar leads?
A   Lead I
B   Lead V4
C   Lead aVL
D   Lead V4R

Answers

1.   A   Ventricular contraction
2.   D   Current flowing away from positive electrode produces a negative waveform
3.   C   Left ventricle
4.   B   Positive
5.   C   Lead V5
6.   A   Time
7.   C   0.06-0.10 seconds
8.   A   Lead I

CHAPTER 4

Systematic Interpretation of EKG

In this chapter

- Steps in basic EKG interpretation

Clinical scenario

It has been a busy morning for student nurse Jean, who is working with her preceptor David in the telemetry unit. One of the patient had tachycardia with the heart rate of 170 bpm and subsequent hypotension and shortness of breath. He was later on transferred to intensive care unit after evaluated by rapid response team. Two other patients went for angiogram and one of them came back after angioplasty. By the time everything was settled, it was 3 O' clock in the afternoon. Jean was somewhat disappointed because even after being with an excellent preceptor like David, she hasn't got any downtime to learn specifics of EKG analysis that David taught her classmates last time. As soon as she got an opportunity, Jean asked David "I know you were quite busy this morning, but I have to ask. Do you have a few minutes to teach me your way of EKG analysis?" Jean continued, "I heard from my classmates that you taught them a systematic method to interpret EKG rhythms that seems to be very helpful for all of them. I have been waiting for my turn to be with you to learn that". "Not a problem. Let me finish this charting on patient just came back from Cath Lab and then we'll talk", David said by scrolling through the computer screen. Once finished, David got up and said "let's go to the other side of nurse's station. It is less crowded over there". Jean started walking with David down the hall. Then he started explaining.

For untrained eyes, an EKG strip is a series of squiggly lines that doesn't tell anything by itself. However, for the trained mind of medical personnel, it is the holy grail of information about someone's heart. Since there is so much information hidden among these wavy lines, at times matters life and death, it is imperative that the person who is reading EKG should do it in a systematic and orderly fashion to avoid any possibility of overlooking vital information. For individuals who are beginning to practice the techniques of EKG interpretation, the systematic assessment may appear cumbersome and tedious. However, by constant practice and experience this technique becomes a second nature.

Steps in EKG Interpretation

1. Determine Rhythm and Regularity

The first and foremost step in evaluating an EKG strip is identifying components of the rhythm. As we mentioned in earlier chapters, normal EKG is a true representation of electrical functions of the heart. Therefore, we should have a P wave that represents channelization of electrical impulse and contraction response of atria in the beginning of each complex. *Presence of P wave* thereby ensures the fact that this *electrical impulse is coming off of the atrium*. We should also see a sequential downward movement of electrical impulse to the next destination, the AV node. As we know, there's going to be a delay in AV node that corresponds an isoelectric line between P wave and QRS complex called PR interval. Then the impulse travels through both ventricles results in depolarization (contraction) and produces a tall QRS complex. After contraction of chambers in response to this electrical impulse, ventricles relax (repolarize) back to their original state and are represented in the EKG as a T wave. There may also be a small U wave that represents late ventricular repolarization and it follows T wave. In order to assess the rhythm, we have to make sure all these waves are present, and they appear in regular intervals and sequence.

Depending on the presence or absence of P wave, rhythm can be classified into atrial and ventricular rhythm. *If a P wave is present before every QRS complex, it represents a rhythm originating above the ventricle.* If there is presence of P wave and it has the same deflection as the QRS complex, mostly it is sinus rhythm. If the P wave is absent, inverted or show up after QRS complex, resulting rhythm is originating from atrio ventricular junction and is called junctional rhythm. If there is no P wave and only QRS complex, then the rhythm is ventricular in origin. During this step, also look for regularity of the rhythm by analyzing P-P and R-R interval. In a *regular rhythm*, these measurements are *constant from beat to beat.*

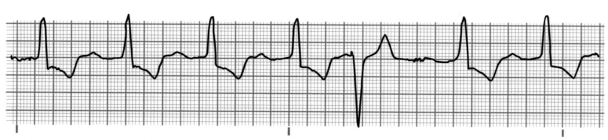

Fig 4.1 Regular rhythm with one irregular beat

In some instances, the rhythm can be regular in most of the part except one extra beat that make the entire rhythm look irregular as shown in Fig 4.1. Therefore, while assessing the regularity of rhythm, we need to evaluate the entire length of available EKG tracing. If we find a premature beat in one section, exclude that area from general assessment so that an accurate interpretation can be made. Most of the time, these isolated premature beats are benign. However, in some situations these premature beats can present at regular intervals such as every other beat or every third beat (bigeminy and trigeminy). At that instance, the rhythm should be classified as *regularly irregular*.

In *completely irregular rhythms*, P-P and R-R measurements will be different from beat to beat as in Fig 4.2. This chaotic rhythm may have *multiple P waves* between each R wave as in the case of Atrial fibrillation. Here, the origin of R waves will be in random. In EKG leads with no R wave and a predominant QS pattern such as Lead V1, S-S interval may be used in place of R-R (Fig 4.3).

Clinical scenario

"Now, let's see how we can calculate the heart rate from a given EKG strip. There are various methods. Some methods are useful when the rhythm is regular, not so fast or not so slow. But when you get in to too fast or too slow or erratic rhythm patterns, you have to rely on more than one method

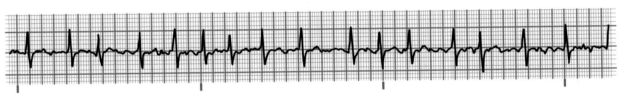

Fig 4.2 Atrial fibrillation (Please note the varying P-P and R-R interval)

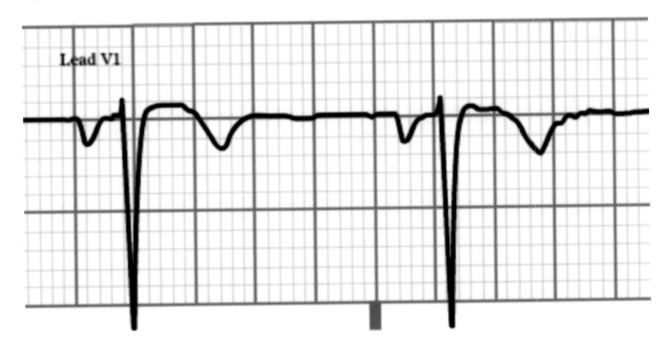

Fig 4.3 Lead V1 with QS pattern instead of usual QRS

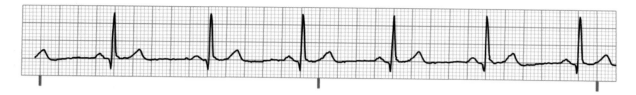

Fig 4.4 Six-second method of calculating rate

to accurately identify the patient's heart rate. Let me grab some rhythm strips from the monitor tech". David got up and reached over the counter to the other side and asked Ben who is the monitor tech. "Hey man, can you please print a strip on umm... say bed four, eleven and eighteen please. It's for me to explain the rate calculation for our nursing student Jean. These patients seem to have heart rhythms qualify for fast, slow and normal pattern". " Give me a minute" Ben replied. " Let me just finish entering this order in the system. I will bring them to you once they get printed". "Okay, Thanks man, appreciate your help" David replied. He then sat down and started explaining to Jean. After couple of minutes, Ben came back with three EKG strips and asked. " You asked for bed four, eleven and eighteen. right? Here they are". David said " Yes... Thanks so much man, how can we survive without you...". " I know, you guys will be perished if I am not here..." Ben said in a sarcastic tone and continued, "Anyway,

go on. I don't want to waste Jean's quality time with you, I will mess with you later". David smiled at Ben and then returned to the strips and laid them over the table. He then pulled out a caliper from his pocket and started explaining.

2. Calculate Rate

While assessing the heart rate, we are more interested in the rate of ventricular contraction than that of atria since ventricles are the main pumping chambers of the heart. Therefore, heart rate is calculated by assessing the *number of QRS complex in 1 min*. The rate of atrial and ventricular contraction is identical in a regular rhythm as there is only one P wave preceding every QRS complex. During irregular rhythms, the rate of atrial contraction is the number of P waves present in 1 min and rate of ventricular contraction is the number of QRS complexes in the same timeframe. There are various methods available for calculation of heart rate from EKG.

1. The Six Second Method

This is the fastest but least reliable method for assessing heart rate. Here, *count the number of QRS complex in a six second EKG strip and multiply by 10* and that will give you heart rate in 60 seconds or 1 min. For example, in a given EKG if there are six QRS complexes within six seconds, according to this method the heart rate will be 6 X 10 = 60 bpm. This method is particularly used for calculating regular rhythms.

Steps in EKG Interpretation

1. Determine the rhythm and regularity
2. Calculate the rate
3. Evaluate P wave
4. Calculate PR interval
5. Analyze QRS complex
6. Examine T wave
7. Calculate QT interval
8. Look for other characteristics

Box 4.1 Steps in EKG interpretation

2. Counting Large Box Method

This method involves memorizing a sequence of numbers and applying it on a given strip. This method relies on the fact that there are 300 large boxes within 1 min strip. Therefore, *counting the number of big boxes between two consecutive R waves and dividing it into 300* will give you the heart rate. You may use the same method on P waves to find atrial rate.

In order to perform this method, we have to find one R wave that is perfectly aligned with the thick line of a large box in the EKG grid and start counting number of large boxes until the next R wave. For example, if there are five large boxes between two R waves, the heart rate will be 300/5 = 60 bpm. For easier calculation, you may memorize the sequence of numbers like 300- 150- 100- 75 - 60- 50 and so on. That means if there are two large blocks between consecutive R waves, heart rate will be 300/2 = 150. If there are three large boxes, heart rate is 300/3 = 100 bpm. So, if you have 10 large boxes between two consecutive R waves, rate is 300/10 = 30. In the given example, there are four large boxes between two consecutive R waves and therefore the rate of contraction is 300/4 = 75 beats per minute.

3. Counting Small Box Method

Similar to the earlier method, it is based on the fact that there are 1500 small boxes in 1 min strip. Therefore, in order to calculate ventricular rate, you may count the number of small boxes between two consecutive R waves and

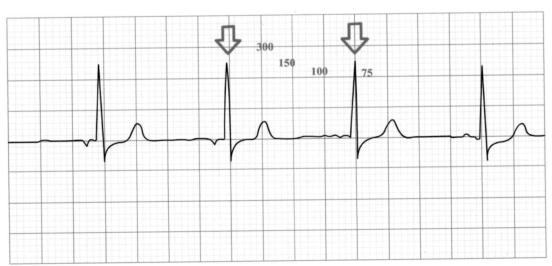

Fig 4.5 Counting large box method

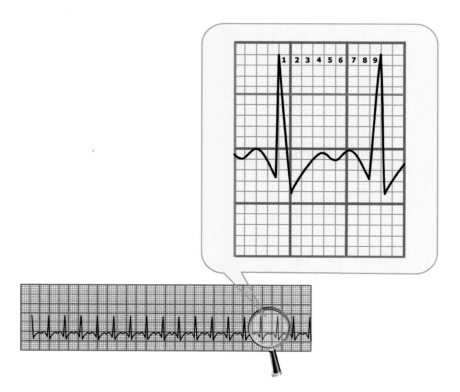

Fig 4.6 Small box counting method

divided into 1500. This method is particularly *useful for fast rhythms*, where it may be hard to align one QRS with thick line of large box. For example, if there are 9 small boxes between two R waves as shown in the picture, heart rate will be 1500/9 = 166 bpm.

Clinical scenario

"*Well, now you know how to assess the heart rate from various strips. After this, I would like you to grab some strips from Ben and calculate the rate and other characteristics. When you practice them, you can retain what you learned. I can also help you on the way if you have any questions*", David said." Absolutely, I love to do that", Jean replied. "Now, let

me explain briefly what else we need to look for in an EKG strip to accurately interpret what is happening with the patient". David said while reaching for a sheet of paper from the stack at the corner.

3. Evaluate P Wave

Check for presence of P wave, their size and shape, variability and presence of one P wave for each QRS complex. Presence of P wave indicates that the rhythm is originating from above the ventricle. In *normal sinus rhythm, there will be one identical P wave before each QRS complex*. In situations where other ectopic foci within the atria produce impulses, the shape of P wave can be varying (wandering pacemaker). If the P wave appears to be inverted, biphasic or following QRS, then the rhythm is junctional. *P waves are absent in pure ventricular rhythms.* It is worth mentioning that some of the fast rhythms like supraventricular tachycardia, *P waves may not be visible* because of the close proximity of two consecutive QRS complexes.

4. Calculate PR Interval

PR interval *is the time taken for the impulse to travel from atria to the ventricle.* Therefore, elongation of PR interval shows additional delay for impulse to travel between the two chambers as seen in various types of heart block. In order to assess PR interval, *count the number of small boxes between the beginning of P wave to the beginning of QRS complex and multiply by 0.4.* Resulting value is the PR interval in seconds. For example, normal PR interval is 3 to 5 small boxes i.e. **0.12-0.20 seconds.** You need to *assess PR interval in multiple areas of the same strip* so that any irregularity in PR interval, which is the hallmark of various types of heart block can be found.

5. Analyze QRS Complex

Count the *number of small boxes starting from the beginning of QRS complex* (i.e. from the end of PR interval) *to the end of S wave and multiply by 0.04.* Normal QRS complex duration is **0.06 - 0.10 seconds.** Look for other characteristics such as the size, symmetry, shape and presence of QRS after each P wave.

6. Evaluate T Wave

Examine the EKG for presence of T waves after each QRS, its shape (upright or inverted), amplitude (normally *not more than 1/2 the size of R wave*), any abnormal appearance (presence of hidden P wave within T wave) and presence of U wave after T waves.

7. Calculate QT Interval

QT interval represents *the time duration of depolarization and repolarization of ventricles.* Again, *count the number of small boxes between beginning of Q wave and end of T wave and multiply by 0.4.* Normal QT interval is between **0.36- 0.44 seconds.**

8. Other Characteristics

Look for other characteristics such as ectopic beats, pauses and any regularity of these events, ST segment changes, dropped beats, presence of multiple P waves for each QRS etc. This time, you essentially put together all the information gathered in previous steps.

Clinical scenario

At the end of the day, Jean finished looking at strips for all of her patients and was able to identify various characteristics of those rhythms. David was there to help her whenever she had any questions. Jean was so happy since she managed to squeeze in some learning time within the hectic twelve-hour shift with David. "I know, you went through a crash course on rhythm analysis today. But keep on practicing. If you use it every day you will never forget. Follow the basic steps no matter how complex the rhythm is". David said. "Sure, I will try to practice rhythm analysis every time I am on the unit. Honestly, now it starts making sense when I look at a rhythm strip. Thanks for your awesome explanations and helping me to learn these techniques" Jean thanked David.

Points to Remember!!!

- Presence of P wave in the beginning of an EKG complex represents an atrial rhythm.
- Junctional rhythms may have inverted, absent or trailing P waves.
- In regular rhythms, P-P and R-R interval are constant from beat to beat.
- In regularly irregular rhythm such as bigeminy or trigeminy, measurements of intervals should be done on regular waveforms.
- In completely irregular rhythms as in atrial fibrillation, P-P and R-R interval varies from beat to beat.
- In regular rhythms, heart rate can be calculated by multiplying the number of QRS complexes within six seconds strip in to 10.
- In order to calculate rate by counting large box method, count the number of large boxes between two constitutive R waves and dividing it into 300.
- For rapid rhythms, count number of small boxes between two adjacent R waves and divide into 1500 gives the heart rate.
- All measurements need to be done in multiple areas of the same strip in order to avoid any possible beat to beat variations affecting the values.
- Presence of P waves with more than one morphology represent origin of impulses from multiple pacemaker sites as in the case of wandering pacemaker.
- In junctional rhythms, there may be inverted, absent or trailing P waves for each QRS complex.
- Normal PR interval is 0.12 to 0.20 seconds and QRS duration is 0.06 to 0.10 seconds.
- Normal QT interval is between 0.36 to 0.44 seconds

Test Your Understanding

1. Which of the following statement regarding an irregular rhythm is true?
A   P-P and R-R intervals are constant from beat to beat
B   P-P and R-R intervals does not match from beat to beat
C   P-P interval is always constant; however, R-R interval varies
D   P-P interval varies with a constant R-R interval

2. The hallmark characteristic of atrial rhythm is _____?
A   Presence of U wave
B   Presence of inverted P wave
C   Presence of biphasic T wave
D   Presence of P wave

3. Which of the following statement is true in measuring intervals on any rhythm strip?
A   All measurements are done on the first beat of the strip
B   All measurements are done on the last beat of the strip
C   All measurements need to be repeated at various beats within the same strip
D   All measurements to be repeated on first and last beat of the strip

4. Which of the following accurately represent calculation of heart rate by counting large box method?
A   Count the number of large boxes between two adjacent R waves and divided into 1500

B   Count the number of small boxes between adjacent R waves and divided in to 300

C   Count the number of large boxes between adjacent R waves and multiply by 10

D   Count the number of large box is between adjacent R waves and divided into 300

5. The best method for calculating heart rate in supraventricular tachycardia is _____?

A   Six seconds strip method

B   Counting small boxes

C   Counting large boxes

D   Counting number of QRS complex in the whole strip

Answers

1.   B   P-P and R-R intervals does not match from beat to beat

2.   D   Presence of P wave

3.   C   All measurements need to be repeated at various beats within the same strip

4.   D   Count the number of large boxes between adjacent R waves and divided into 300

5.   B   Counting small boxes

PART 2

UNDERSTANDING ARRHYTHMIAS

CHAPTER 5

SA Nodal Rhythms

In this chapter

- Normal sinus rhythm
- Sinus arrhythmia
- Sinus bradycardia
- Sinus tachycardia
- Sinus arrest
- Sino atrial exit block
- Inappropriate sinus tachycardia
- Sick sinus syndrome

Clinical scenario

It was an unusually quiet afternoon in the Memorial hospital emergency room. Ben, newly graduated emergency room RN noticed that the triage area was almost empty, and the ambulance bay was unusually clear compared to everyday frenzy. He walked up to the reception area where he overheard the chatter on the radio from emergency medical personnel about a patient with head injury on the way to ER with ETA 2 minutes. Within few minutes, paramedics wheeled in with a morbidly obese male patient on the gurney who had blood all over his shirt and a bandage on his forehead. Ben went and helped Mira who is another ER nurse in placing the patient on monitor and setting up IV lines. According to the paramedics, the patient felt dizzy at the mall and fell down a small stairwell and hit his head. Patient never lost consciousness and there were no witnessed seizure episodes. Within 5 minutes, patient was taken to CT scan. Couple of hours later, finally when patient was transferred to ICU, Ben went and asked Mira, "Hey Mira, I heard the ER resident calling cardiologist on call for your guy with head injury. Why was he calling the cardiologist instead of neurologist for a patient who passed out and came with a head injury?" "Oh, it was because the patient appeared to have sick sinus syndrome that caused him to collapse". Mira replied. " I think I heard about sick sinus syndrome before. Can you please explain little bit?, Ben said. "No problem, this is the best time because I am about to close the chart on Mr. Hamilton as he got transferred to ICU. Let me show you the EKG strip that documented sick sinus." Mira said while clicking on different tabs on the computer screen. " Look at these rhythm Ben", Mira continued, "Here we have a strip where patient had his heart rate at 130's and here is one with rate around 30 with long pauses, all within one hour. Patient was actually feeling dizzy and his pressure dropped when his rate was at 30. Dr. Jacobson put in a transvenous pacemaker for the patient before transferring him to ICU. He was a classic case of tachy-brady syndrome". Ben asked, " So... why did that happen? How come patient has that much variability in his heart rate?". "Well, if you want to understand the whole concept, you need to know various types of rhythms originating from the sinus node. I hope another ambulance is not rolling in with someone for me. Let me close this chart and then will explain" Mira said and walked towards the corner cabinet with a folder in her hand. After few minutes, Mira came back and started explaining to Ben. " Okay, let's look at various types of rhythms from the sinus node".

These are cardiac rhythms originating from the SA node, which is the natural pacemaker of the heart. All of these rhythms will have the characteristic *uniform P waves before each QRS complexes*. These rhythms can be normal or abnormal such as normal sinus rhythm, sinus tachycardia, sinus bradycardia, sinus arrest etc.

Normal Sinus Rhythm

Normal sinus rhythm occurs when an impulse originates in SA node and then proceed to AV node, which then progress down to the ventricles through normal pathways resulting in a normal P and QRS complex.

Basic characteristics are

Rhythm:	Atrial: regular, Ventricular: regular
Rate:	60 to 100 bpm
P wave:	normal and uniform
PR interval:	0.12 - 0.20 sec (within normal limits)
QRS complex:	0.06- 0.10 Sec (within normal limits)
T wave:	normal and uniform
QT interval:	0.36 - 0.44 Sec (within normal limits)

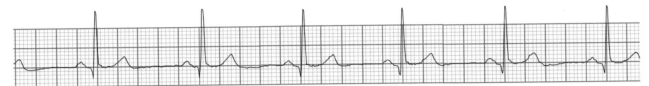

Fig 5.1 Normal sinus rhythm

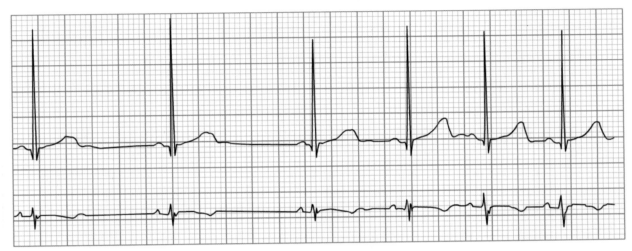

Fig 5.2 Sinus arrhythmia

Sinus Arrhythmia

In sinus arrhythmia, the heart rate stays within normal limits however, the rhythm will be irregular. There will be *waxing and waning of heart rate in response to respiration*. As mentioned in chapter 1, sinus arrhythmia is the result of **vagal control** over the heart. It is assumed that during expiration there is a natural vagal stimulation and is responsible for slowing down of the heart rate. This is commonly seen in athletes, children and patients with sleep apnea.

Basic characteristics are

Rhythm:	irregular and corresponds with respiratory cycle
Rate:	*rate increases on inspiration and decreases with expiration*
P wave:	uniform size and configuration

PR interval:	may vary slightly, but remain within normal limits
QRS complex:	normal configuration
T wave:	within normal limits
QT interval:	may vary slightly between beats, but stays within normal

Clinical significance: there is *no pathophysiologic significant and no treatment* is needed.

Sinus Bradycardia

This rhythm is characterized by sinus rhythm with *heart rate below 60*.

Basic characteristics are

Rhythm:	regular
Rate:	*less than 60 bpm*
P wave:	uniform size and configuration

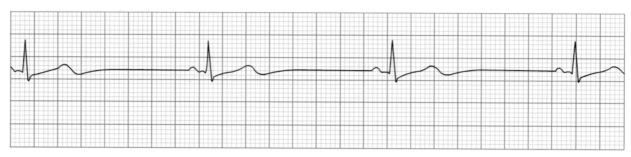

Fig 5.3 Sinus bradycardia

PR interval: within normal limits and constant

QRS complex: normal

T wave: uniform shape

QT interval: normal

Clinical significance: Brady arrhythmia can result in hemodynamic compromise and symptoms such as *syncope, chest pain, premature beats, ventricular tachycardia* etc. Mostly, sinus bradycardia is benign however, if the rate goes below 40 bpm, patient may become symptomatic. Sinus bradycardia is normal in athletes because of their conditioning of the heart.

Etiology: Etiology of SA node dysfunction causing brady arrhythmia can be

(1) **Extrinsic factors** such as influence of drugs (e.g. digitalis), autonomic nervous system response (vagal stimulations from vomiting or straining for bowel movement), hypothyroidism, sleep apnea, hypothermia, hypoxia, increased intracranial pressure (Cushing's response) or endotracheal suctioning etc.

(2) **Intrinsic factors** are degeneration and fibrosis of SA nodal areas from coronary artery disease, pericarditis, myocarditis, rheumatic heart disease, systemic lupus erythematosus (SLE), genetic disorders etc.

Management: *No treatment is necessary if the patient is asymptomatic and the rate stays close to 60 bpm.* If the patient becomes symptomatic, emergency treatment involves administration of Atropine. Once hemodynamically stable, identify the underlying reason for sinus bradycardia. In emergent situations, a temporary pacemaker may be helpful. Once sinus node dysfunction is confirmed, patient may benefit from permanent pacemaker implantation.

Sinus Tachycardia

Sinus tachycardia involves accelerated firing of SA node with a rate greater than 100 beats per minute.

Basic characteristics are

Rhythm: regular

Rate: *greater than 100 beats per minute* (rarely above 160)

P wave: normal size and configuration. However, as the rate increases it may be hidden in T waves

PR interval: shorter because of the fast heart rate

QRS complex: constant and within normal limits

T wave: constant and within normal limits

QT interval: mostly shorter

Clinical significance: Commonly, sinus tachycardia is considered as a *symptom of an underlying pathophysiologic process* and therefore, attention

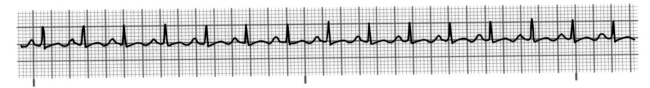

Fig 5.4 Sinus tachycardia

should be directed towards finding primary cause rather than treating it right away. Rarely, patients can have so-called 'Inappropriate sinus tachycardia' (IST). Sinus tachycardia is a *sign of cardiac compensation* to maintain tissue perfusion in the event of hypovolemia, sepsis, hyperthyroidism, heart failure or other forms of sympathetic stimulation. Because of the increased heart rate, this rhythm may considerably increase myocardial oxygen demand and can precipitate heart failure and anginal symptoms.

Inappropriate Sinus Tachycardia (IST)

Unlike in regular sinus tachycardia, there may not be an identifiable underlying factor that causes tachyarrhythmia during this event. IST remains largely a 'diagnosis of exclusion'. In these patients, heart rate increases either spontaneously or after physical activity *disproportionate to their effort level*. Frequent incidence of IST may produce symptoms like chest pain, headache and GI upset, and can be disabling for the patient.

In many patients, the symptoms can be seen *after a viral illness* and *spontaneously recover* in *9 to 12 months* period. For symptomatic patients, treatment choices include *maintaining hydration* and *beta-blockers*. In severely symptomatic individuals, permanent pacemaker implantation and subsequent *radiofrequency ablation of SA node* is an option.

Box 5.1 Inappropriate Sinus Tachycardia

Management: As mentioned earlier, investigation should be directed towards *identifying and treating underlying disease process* that is causing sinus tachycardia. If sinus tachycardia itself is causing hemodynamic compromise, pharmacologic agents like beta-blockers, calcium channel blockers, adenosine or digoxin may be helpful. Patient should be monitored for signs of decreased cardiac output and impaired left ventricular function in the event of profound sinus tachycardia. Supportive measures with administration of oxygen may be helpful in preventing myocardial oxygen depletion.

Sinus Arrest

In this type of rhythm, a normal sinus rhythm is interrupted by *prolonged failure of SA node to initiate an impulse* resulting in *complete missing of PQRST* complex.

Basic characteristics are

Rhythm:	regular except missing complex (pause)
Rate:	usually within normal limits; however, length and frequency of pauses may lead to bradycardia
P wave:	*normal except during pause with missing PQRST complex*. The P wave may retain its uniform shape

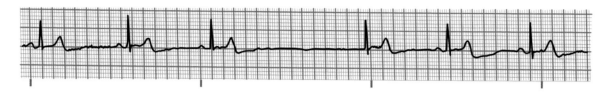

Fig 5.5 Sinus arrest

as before depending on whether SA node or other ectopic pacemakers regain function after the pause.

PR interval: within normal limits; however, may be different in following EKG complex depends on the origin of impulse.

QRS complex: one complete QRS complex will be absent during the pause. Following QRS may assume its shape depending on whether it is SA nodal rhythm or escape beat.

T wave: normal except during arrest where there is no T wave. Again, depending on the site of origin of impulse, it may be normal or abnormal in the following beats.

QT interval: same as in T wave; absent during pause and normal or abnormal in the following beats

Clinical significance: patients are asymptomatic when the length of pause is shorter; however, longer pause can create hemodynamic compromise and may need intervention.

Etiology: Most common causes for sinus arrest are *ischemia affecting SA node*, *effect of SA nodal blocking drugs* (e.g. beta blockers) and *excessive vagal tone*.

Management: depends on the underlying reasons and presenting symptoms. Treatment options are same as that of sinus bradycardia.

Sinus Exit Block

In this situation, sinus node fires impulse however, it doesn't generate a subsequent QRST complex because of the lack of conduction down the pathway. Unlike in sinus arrest, this is a *conduction disturbance rather than problem with cell automaticity*. There may be one or more P waves get blocked, leading to a pause in rhythm. Interestingly, the rhythm regains to normal sinus rhythm as before. The most distinguishable character between sinus exit block and sinus arrest is that *the pause will be a multiplier of R-R interval*. For example, if there are two non-conducted P waves, the length of pause will be two times R-R interval. This is because, unlike in sinus arrest where an escape pacemaker takes over impulse formation immediately after the pause due to the lack of SA node activity; here, the normal SA node impulse start propagating leading to normal sinus rhythm.

Basic characteristics are

Rhythm: regular except during pause
Rate: usually within normal limits; however, bradycardia if length of pause is long

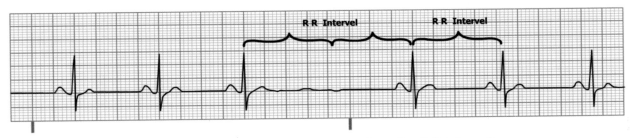

Fig 5.6 Sinus exit block (Note that the length of pause is two times the R-R interval)

P wave:	periodically absent during pause, otherwise normal
PR interval:	normal except during the pause
QRS complex:	within normal limits; missing during pause
T wave:	absent during the pause

Other characteristics: *length of pause is a multiplier of R-R interval*

Clinical significance: only if the length of pause is longer, it may cause hemodynamic compromise or subjective symptoms. Treat as if sinus bradycardia.

"Okay, so far you have seen various types of rhythms originating from the sinus node. Now let's see what exactly sick sinus syndrome or tachy-brady syndrome is? In order to understand the mechanism, you should learn some intrinsic control systems within our heart" Mira explained.

Sick Sinus Syndrome (SSS)

Just as the name implies, sick sinus syndrome (SSS) is a clinical condition with *sickness of the natural pacemaker of the heart*. This SA node dysfunction can be caused by degeneration and fibrous replacement of SA node tissue resulting from inferior wall MI, pericarditis, myocarditis, rheumatic heart disease, SLE or some genetic mutations. Failure of SA node to generate impulses leads to activation of ectopic pacemakers within the atria and resultant tachyarrhythmia mostly in the form of atrial fibrillation or flutter.

Cardiac cells have an innate property called override suppression phenomena. The automaticity of pacemaker cells diminishes after they are stimulated by an impulse at a higher frequency as in atrial fibrillation. Even after the ectopic foci stop firing, SA node cells remain dormant for little longer. This leads to creation of a long pause in the EKG. Absence of cardiac output during this time can cause clinical symptoms. *The time taken for SA node to reclaim its pacemaker function* after the end of tachyarrhythmia is called sinus node recovery time. In patients with sick sinus syndrome, this recovery time maybe longer than usual. If the period of asystole is significantly long, patients can have loss of consciousness. As the heart rhythm varies between tachycardia and bradycardia, it is also called 'tachy-brady syndrome'.

Basic characteristics are

Rhythm:	irregular with sinus pauses. May have sinus arrest, sinus

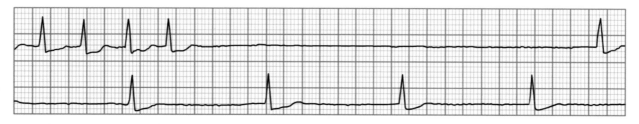

Fig 5.7 Sick sinus syndrome with pause (Note the sinus node recovery time after tachycardia leading to a long pause)

exit block or long pause following termination of tachycardia.

Rate: alternate between slow and fast pace

Management: depending on the presentation of cardiac rhythm, management may differ.

In general, for bradycardia causing profound symptoms, **permanent pacemaker implantation** is warranted. As far as the tachycardia component is concerned, management varies depending on the type of rhythm. If the patient has underlying atrial fibrillation or flutter, various drugs or radiofrequency catheter ablation may be helpful. In the event the patient has chronic atrial fibrillation, he or she may need thromboembolic prevention by use of oral anticoagulants like Coumadin or Dabigatran. In many instances, patient may require permanent pacemaker to treat bradycardia and rate control agents like beta-blockers and calcium channel blocker for tachycardia.

Clinical scenario

"Well, now it makes sense why the Resident was calling cardiologist for that patient. Does he need permanent pacemaker?" Ben asked. "May or may not. The cardiologist will first evaluate him for any reversible causes for bradycardia like any medications. If he continued to have pauses despite any such treatable pathology, he may end up in receiving a pacer. At that point they can treat him with medications for his fast heart rhythm without having the fear of making him bradycardic. Mr. Hamilton is going to be admitted to the hospital for a few days for evaluation." Mira said. "Thank you so much for your explanations. I learned a lot. I think it's almost time for change of shift and looks like you survived without another admit. I will let you finish things before your shift ends. Again, thanks so much". "You are most welcome, oh! I see you are swing shift today. So basically, stuck here for now, sorry about that" Mira chuckled. "That's ok, at least I can learn all these interesting things from you guys when I am here. Have a nice evening. Will see you tomorrow". Ben said. "Okay, see you tomorrow. Have a good evening. I am going to clock out in few minutes" Mira replied.

Points to Remember!!!

- All SA nodal rhythms have a uniform P wave before each QRS complex.
- In sinus arrhythmia, there is waxing and waning of heart rate in response to respiration.
- Sinus arrhythmia is an example of vagal control over the heart.
- Sinus bradycardia can be caused by extrinsic factors (drugs, vagal stimulation, hypothermia, hypoxia) or intrinsic factors (degradation of SA node, pericarditis, myocarditis, rheumatic heart disease).
- Administration of atropine and temporary or permanent pacemaker implantation are the treatment for sinus bradycardia.
- Mostly, sinus tachycardia is a symptom of an underlying pathology than a disease by itself.
- Tachycardia disproportionate to the effort level is called inappropriate sinus tachycardia.
- Beta-blockers, calcium channel blockers, adenosine and digoxin are the possible treatment options for sinus tachycardia.
- Sinus arrest is caused by prolonged delay in initiation of impulse from SA node.
- Excessive vagal tone, ischemia or fibrosis of SA node and effect of nodal blocking drugs are the usual causes for sinus arrest.
- Unlike in sinus arrest, during sinus exit block there is impulse production from the SA node. However, there is failure of impulse conduction down the system.
- Major differentiation of the pause caused by sinus exit block is that the pause is a multiplier of R-R interval.

- In sick sinus syndrome, there is prolonged sinus node recovery time after tachycardia event; leading to a pause.
- Because of override suppression phenomena of cardiac cells, they respond only to the fastest stimuli available to them irrespective of its origin. This is the reason for excitation of heart by fast ectopic pacemakers.
- Permanent pacemaker implantation for management of bradycardia along with nodal blocking agents for treatment of tachycardia is the mode of therapy for tachy-brady syndrome.

Test Your Understanding

1. Which of the following represent the most distinguishable character of sinus arrhythmia?
A   Heart rate below 50 bpm
B   Heart rate above 150 bpm
C   Increasing and decreasing heart rate with respiration
D   Presence of intermittent pause

2. Treatment for sinus bradycardia includes _____?
A   Beta-blockers
B   Digoxin
C   Atropine
D   Verapamil

3. Which of the following is not a treatment option for inappropriate sinus tachycardia?
A   Beta-blockers
B   Radiofrequency ablation
C   Permanent pacemaker
D   Atropine

4. Which of the following statement is true for the pause during sinus exit block?

A   Length of the pause is half of RR interval

B   Length of the pause is a multiplier of PR interval

C   Length of pause is a multiplier of R-R interval

D   Length of pause does not correlate with R-R interval

5. Which of the following is a true definition of override protection phenomena of cardiac cells?

A   Cardiac cells respond to the fastest stimuli available to them irrespective of its source

B   Cardiac cells respond to the fastest stimuli only if it is from SA node

C   Cardiac cells respond to the slowest available stimuli irrespective of its strength

D   Cardiac cells respond to the slowest available stimuli only if it is strong enough

Answers

1.   C   Increasing and decreasing heart rate with respiration

2.   C   Atropine

3.   D   Atropine

4.   C   Length of pause is a multiplier of R-R interval

5.   A   Cardiac cells respond to the fastest stimuli available to them irrespective of its source

CHAPTER 6

Atrial Dysrhythmia

In this chapter

- Premature atrial complex
- Atrial tachycardia
- Paroxysmal atrial tachycardia
- Multifocal atrial tachycardia
- Atrial flutter
- Atrial fibrillation

Clinical scenario

Ryan is orienting with Jane in ICU and are going to assume care of Mr. Smith who is admitted with tachycardia and hypotension. According to the Night shift RN, he is going to the cath lab for radiofrequency ablation today. Once they finished with report, Jane said " Okay Ryan, since Mr. Smith is going to the cath lab, let's make sure all his pre-procedural orders are finished. We need to prioritize our day." Jane and Ryan went through the patient's chart and made sure the patient has all the preparations including consent, patent IV lines etc. are in place. When Jane and Ryan went to Mr. Smith's room to change the heparin bag that was hanging, his daughter Shelly asked "I wasn't here when the cardiologist talked to my dad about the procedure. Can you explain to me what exactly are they going to do? My dad cannot give me a complete picture. He is saying the doctor told him he is going to make some road blocks within the heart". "Yes, he's correct", Jane replied while helping Ryan to hook up new heparin infusion bag." I'm more than happy to explain to you what the procedure is. Your dad has an abnormal heart rhythm called atrial flutter. During this particular rhythm, the upper chamber of the heart beats faster than the lower chamber due to the presence of some electrical short-circuit within the heart. In the Cath Lab, Dr. Hansen is going to identify these abnormal pathways and interrupt them by burning the inner surface of the heart with heat generated from high-frequency current. These burned areas act as road blocks for the electricity from traveling through the cyclic pathway and create repetitive contractions of the chamber". "So, my dad going to have open heart surgery?" Shelly asked with a frantic look on her face. Jane quickly replied, 'Oh, no... absolutely not. The entire procedure is going to be through a small needle hole created in the artery or vein at his groin area. There is no incision involved except having needles slightly bigger than the one used for IV access in his hand. After the procedure, they will remove everything and all he will have is some prick marks in both groin. They can insert all sorts of equipment and work with them through the small holes. Normally, if all goes well your dad would be able to go home tomorrow". "That's awesome, it's amazing how much they can do nowadays in the field of medicine without cutting anybody open. Thanks for this wonderful explanation. I'm very much relieved. I was so worried about my dad when he called me and said he is going to have a heart procedure. I was at work yesterday and couldn't be here. Now I'm glad that I talk you beforehand, otherwise I would have been great stress during the whole day ", Shelly said. "You'll be seeing Dr. Hansen after the procedure. He usually comes out and talk to the family once he is done at the Cath Lab. When Mr. Smith is going to Cath Lab, I'll let you know where to wait for Dr. Hansen", Jane said. "Thank you so much", Shelly replied by extending her hands for shake hands with Jane. "You're welcome. I will let you know after talking to the Cath Lab what time he is scheduled to go for the procedure. I expect him to go around nine o'clock, but I will confirm it and let you know. Is there anything else I can do for both of you before I leave?" Jane asked. "No, nothing now. You've been very helpful. Again, thanks for the care of my dad and explaining everything for me", Shelly replied. "Not a problem. Okay, then I will be back later. But let me know if there is anything you guys need", Jane said while walking out of the room with Ryan. Once back in the nurse's station Ryan said, "that was a very good explanation you gave to the patient and family about ablation procedure. I'm sure that took care of a lot of her anxiety. When you get a chance, can you please explain to me a little bit more about atrial flutter and fibrillation? I read about them in the past, but has trouble figuring out in the actual EKG rhythm strip". "No problem, we will try to talk about this during the course of the day. I think it is a perfect day to talk about heart rhythms because both of our patients have abnormal heart rhythms. In general, most of these abnormal *rhythms like atrial flutter, fibrillation etc. are due to extra beats within the heart. I'll give you some basics, let's go over to the telemetry station. Let me take this chair with me", Jane replied after getting up and pushing her chair towards the rhythm monitor at the corner of the nurse's station.*

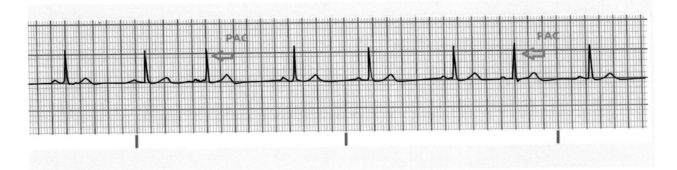

Fig 6.1 Premature atrial contraction

These rhythm disturbances are originating from *ectopic foci within atria other than SA node.* Atrial dysrhythmia can be either isolated and benign as in **premature atrial complex** (PAC) or sustained and irregular that causes hemodynamic compromise like **atrial fibrillation.** Either way, these rhythms carry a *P wave,* which may get buried in the neighboring QRS if rate is high and *a narrow QRS complex* except in selected situations with the presence of aberrant conduction systems.

Premature Atrial Complexes (PAC)

PAC's are formed when an ectopic focus within the atria generate a premature impulse, which either conducted down through the AV node or die down within atria itself. Depending on the timing of this impulse, it may or may not show in the EKG as a distinct wave. For example, if the atrial premature beat originates way early in the cardiac cycle, it may get buried in the QRS complex. If the impulse happens later in the cardiac cycle, PAC can generate a *ventricular contraction that is out of sync* with the rest of the rhythm. Then it will be characterized by a *different shaped P wave.* Sometimes this P wave can be hidden within the T wave of previous QRS complex and thereby causing a *distorted T wave.* Therefore, whenever there is a T wave that is deformed with subsequent normal QRS complex and normal T wave, it raises the suspicion of a PAC.

Basic characteristics are

Rhythm:	normal except during PAC
Rate:	usually within normal limits
P wave:	deformed P during PAC
QRS complex:	normal
T wave:	usually normal unless a P wave hides within it.

QT interval: normal during underlying rhythm; varies if T wave is distorted

Clinical significance: Occasional PACs are completely benign. Once they become more frequent, may cause subjective symptoms such as **palpitations**. Frequent PACs are often prelude to atrial tachycardia or fibrillation. Recurrent PACs can be treated with *Calcium channel blockers*, *digitalis* or *beta-blockers*.

Clinical scenario

After finishing the morning routine, Jane and Ryan sat together at the nurse's station to do documentation for both of their patients. Once finished, they continued the discussion about atrial rhythms. Jane said, "Now, before we go into more details about atrial flutter and fibrillation, let's look at the rhythm strip of Mrs. Garcia who is our next patient", Jane continued while grabbing the mouse and clicking through EKG rhythms in the computer. "Here, look at this strip for Mrs. Garcia. It happened around four o'clock this morning. As you heard from the night nurse during report, Mrs. Garcia had episodes of palpitation early morning. I bet this coincides with her symptoms. This is a classic example of multifocal atrial tachycardia" Jane said by handing over the strip to Ryan. After looking at the strip Ryan asked, "hay Jane, you said the rhythm is multifocal atrial tachycardia, but here it says on the top as supraventricular tachycardia. Are they

the same?" "No, not really". Jane replied. "Let's look at the specifics of atrial tachycardia".

Atrial Tachycardia

These rhythms can be generally named as **Supraventricular tachycardia** (SVT) as all of them *originate above the level of ventricle*. Common forms of atrial tachycardia are **Paroxysmal atrial tachycardia** (PAT) and **Multifocal atrial tachycardia** (MAT) or so-called '**wandering pacemaker**'. These rhythms are characterized by an *atrial rate of 150 to 250 bpm*. Physiologically, these accelerated atrial rhythms diminish '*atrial kick*' that is responsible for approximately 30% of ventricular filling. This may eventually affect cardiac output.

Paroxysmal Atrial Tachycardia (PAT)

Characterized by *sudden onset of three or more beats* of *narrow complex tachycardia*, usually originate with a premature atrial contraction. These rhythms last only for a short duration and is called '**paroxysmal**'. It resembles sinus tachycardia however, the characteristic *initiating PAC* is visible here.

Basic characteristics are

Rhythm: underlying rhythm is regular; interrupted by tachycardia which itself is regular.

Rate: 150 to 250 bpm

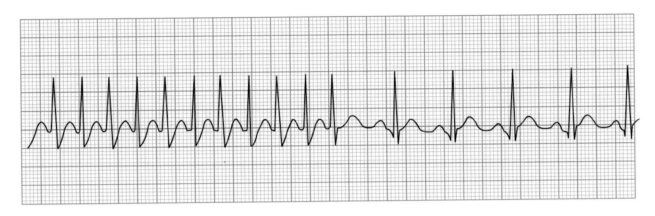

Fig 6.2 Paroxysmal atrial tachycardia converting to sinus rhythm

P wave: uniform shape in underlying rhythm; however, different shaped or absent in tachycardia because it buried under neighboring T wave.

PR interval: within normal limits and constant in underlying rhythm; unidentifiable or shorter during tachycardia

QRS complex: narrow throughout the rhythm

T wave: normal during underlying rhythm; however, distorted in tachycardia.

QT interval: normal during underlying rhythm, shorter in tachycardia.

Clinical significance: Depending on the length of atrial tachycardia, patients may have symptoms ranging from mere palpitation to serious hemodynamic compromise. *Isolated PACs are perfectly normal.*

Etiology: Origin of atrial tachycardia may trace back to problems with *automaticity* or *re-entry* of atrial impulses like in the case of other atrial arrhythmias. Hypoxia, hypocalcemia, Digoxin toxicity, increased vagal tone, cardiomyopathy etc. are the cause of atrial arrhythmias.

Management: Strategy for management of PAC is based on *the length of tachyarrhythmia* and the *extent of symptoms.* Isolated PACs doesn't need any treatment and are benign. However, symptomatic tachycardia needs medications like *beta-blockers, digoxin* or *calcium channel blockers.* Avoidance of stimuli such as *caffeine* or *cigarette* smoking is also important. Rate control in acute situations can be achieved by administration of adenosine or application of vagal maneuvers like carotid sinus massage or coughing. Seriously ill patients may need direct current cardioversion for converting them back to sinus rhythm.

Multifocal Atrial Tachycardia (MAT)

This rhythm is also known as Wandering pacemaker, characterized by *more than one shaped P wave.* During this event, impulses are originating from multiple atrial ectopic foci and hence, different morphology of P wave. Usually *more than three identifiable types of P waves* can be seen.

Basic characteristics are

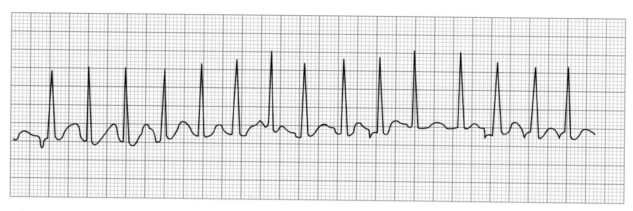

Fig 6.3 Multifocal atrial tachycardia

Rhythm:	irregular
Rate:	usually between 100 to 150 bpm
P wave:	*at least three different morphology*
PR interval:	slightly varies from beat to beat
QRS complex:	within normal limits
T wave:	not uniform
QT interval:	may or may not be measurable

Clinical significance: multifocal atrial tachycardia is mostly seen in patients with significant lung disease like **chronic obstructive pulmonary disease** (**COPD**).

Management: Treatment should be directed towards improving underlying disease for long-term management. For rate control, *calcium channel blockers* like **Verapamil** may be helpful. In patients with *no left ventricular dysfunction* or *coronary artery disease*, pharmacologic agents like **Flecainide** or **Propafenone** may be useful.

Clinical scenario

"Well, now I see that P waves are all different shaped in this rhythm. As you said I can identify three distinct shape P waves. So, this is a case of wandering pacemaker.

I also remember reading the patient's list of diagnosis. Chronic obstructive pulmonary disease was one of them", Ryan said. "You're right", Jane replied and then continued. "She does have COPD and is on home oxygen therapy. You may also see that she is on Cardizem- a calcium channel blocker like verapamil- IV drip for rate control". "Yes, I do". Ryan said by flipping through the medication administration record for Mrs. Garcia. "Now, let's look into the rhythm strip for Mr. Smith. He is constantly in atrial flutter with fixed conduction block", Jane said while grabbing another rhythm strip from the printer. "You may see the characteristic P waves that looks like the teeth of a saw", Jane said by pointing the P wave pattern in the strip with her pen. "Yes, I do see the pattern. it is interesting", Ryan replied. Jane continued, "Let me explain to you bit more about this rhythm".

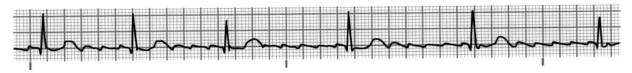

Fig 6.4 Atrial flutter with characteristic saw tooth flutter waves

Atrial Flutter

It is a form of supraventricular tachycardia with an atrial rate of *250 to 400 bpm*. An aberrant pathway causing re-entry of the impulse usually generates this type of rhythm, leading to recurrent atrial depolarization. The most characteristic pattern of atrial flutter is the 'saw tooth' shaped P waves called flutter waves. Because of the inherent safety mechanism within AV node, many of these impulses terminated at the level of AV node leading to 2:1 or 4:1 conduction ratio in the ventricle. Even if there is 2:1 block exists, ventricles may be firing up to 150 bpm and can create serious hemodynamic compromise.

Basic characteristics are

Rhythm:	regular or irregular depending on AV nodal conduction pattern.
Rate:	atrial rate of 250 to 400 bpm; ventricular rate usually 1/2 or 1/4 of atrial rate depend on the conduction ratio.
P wave:	characteristic P wave in atrial flutter is called *flutter wave*. These flutter waves have unique 'saw tooth' appearance and are very regular. There may be two or more flutter waves between two QRS complex.
PR interval:	not measurable because of multiple flutter waves between QRS.
QRS complex:	usually narrow and within normal limits.
T wave:	mostly unidentifiable because of the flutter waves.
QT interval:	indiscernible

Clinical significance: Atrial flutter is common in patients with *congenital heart disease, coronary atherosclerosis, valvular heart disease* etc. If untreated, this tachyarrhythmia can significantly *increase myocardial workload*, leading to *left ventricular dysfunction* and possible ischemia in presence of co-morbid conditions. Because of the pooling of blood within the atria secondary to tachycardia, *risk of thromboembolic event is high*.

Management: Pharmacologic agents like *calcium channel blockers* (**Diltiazem, Verapamil**), *Digoxin* and *beta-blockers* may be helpful in controlling ventricular rate by slowing AV nodal conduction. Electrical cardioversion after adequate anticoagulation may provide long-term solution.

Most common atrial flutter circuit is located in the right atrium around tricuspid valve annulus. This pathway facilitates re-entry of impulses back to right atrium causing repeated depolarization. Knowledge of this anatomic location of re-entry circuit is extremely important in the treatment of atrial flutter with *radiofrequency ablation*. During RF ablation, an *electrical roadblock is created in the circuit* leading to termination of its re-entry.

"Now… just have a look at this rhythm. Can you tell me what you are seeing here", Jane asked Ryan while pointing her pen to the central telemetry monitor. Ryan said, "Hum… I do see QRS complexes. For sure it is not regular. Where is the P wave? I don't see it." "Good observation, you are right. There is no P wave and the rhythm is irregular in this pattern", Jane replied. She then continued, "what you just said is a characteristic of a heart rhythm called atrial fibrillation".

Atrial Fibrillation

It is the most common sustained atrial arrhythmia characterized by *rapid, disorganized* and *irregular atrial activation,* most likely from *multiple ectopic foci.* This multi-center stimulation of atria results in disorganized depolarization and practically a '*trembling*' or '*vibrating*' movement of the chamber. During this event, AV node acts as a natural protective mechanism for the ventricles. It blocks most of these erratic impulses and only allows smaller number of them to conduct down to the ventricles, leading to **controlled ventricular response (CVR)**. However, in some instances, AV node allows most of these fibrillatory waves to pass down to ventricles leading to **rapid ventricular response (RVR)**. There are uneven baseline fibrillatory waves and irregular QRS complexes seen in EKG.

Basic characteristics are

Rhythm:	irregularly irregular (both atria and ventricle)
Rate:	Atrial - *above 400 bpm*, no distinguishable uniform P waves seen.

Ventricle- depending on the conduction block at AV node, it may be fast (greater than 100 in RVR) or slow (less than 100 in CVR)

P wave:	*no distinct P waves*, only fibrillatory waves
PR interval:	not measurable
QRS complex:	narrow
T wave:	mostly indiscernible
QT interval:	not measurable

Clinical significance: Important clinical significances of atrial fibrillation are (1) **loss of atrial contractility** (2) **inappropriately fast ventricular response** (3) **loss of atrial appendage contractility** leading *to risk of clots formation* and subsequent *thromboembolic event.*

Interestingly, in some patients with atrial fibrillation, **lead V1** shows flutter wave pattern rather than chaotic fibrillatory waves because the **crista terminalis**. This is a thick and smooth surfaced portion of the heart muscle at the opening of right atrial appendage that blocks fibrillatory waves from conducting to lead V1. Therefore, what lead V1 sees is only atrial activity on lateral aspect of right ventricle.

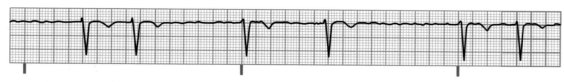

Fig 6.5 **Atrial fibrillation**

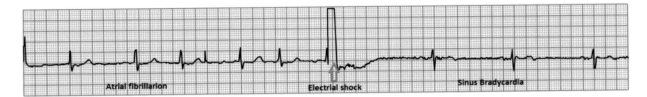

Fig 6.6 Cardioversion of Atrial fibrillation to Sinus rhythm

Many patients are asymptomatic however, palpitation, irregular pulse, hypertension, exercise intolerance, fatigue and pulmonary congestion are seen at times. In some occasions, patients will present with severe dizziness or syncope. This commonly happens in **paroxysmal** (short lasting) **atrial fibrillation,** where sinus node recovery time is unusually longer after termination of atrial fibrillation leading to short period of practical **asystole**.

Classification of Atrial Fibrillation

Paroxysmal	Recurrent episodes that self-terminate in *less than seven days*
Persistent	Recurrent episodes that last *more than seven days*
Permanent	Ongoing *long-term episode*

Box 6.1 Classification of Atrial fibrillation

Management: Aggressive management of atrial fibrillation is done by the use of **direct current** (DC) **cardioversion** if hemodynamic compromise is present. Otherwise treatment goals are (1) **rate control** (2) **prevention of thromboembolic event** (3) **rhythm control**.

1. **Rate Control**: In order to control ventricular response; *beta-blockers*, *calcium channel blockers* (non-dihydropyridines e.g. Diltiazem, Verapamil) and *digoxin* are useful.

2. **Prevention of Thromboembolic Event**: Immediate and long-term anticoagulation is extremely important in preventing thrombotic events like **pulmonary embolism** or **cerebrovascular accident**. Intravenous *heparin* or *low molecular weight heparin* (Enoxaparin) can be used in acute phase. **Coumadin** and **Dabigatran** (Pradaxa) are agents of choice for long-term anticoagulation. Risk of thromboembolism in the event of atrial fibrillation is increased by coexisting factors such as *congestive heart failure, hypertension, advanced age, diabetes mellitus and history of stroke* (known as **CHADS2** Score). **Aspirin** can be useful in patients with a low risk for clot formation.

3. **Rhythm Control**: Atrial fibrillation in and by itself is not dangerous as many other ventricular tachyarrhythmia. As long as the rhythm is not affecting hemodynamics, immediate management is directed towards *rate control and prevention of thromboembolism*. However, in long run, *rhythm control* with conversion back to sinus rhythm with the use of chemical or electrical cardioversion is indicated. Most common anti-arrhythmic agents are **Amiodarone, Dronedarone** (Multaq), **Flecainide** and **Sotalol**. For further details of these drugs, please refer to chapter 14

Clinical scenario

By the time the shift finished, Jane and Ryan had discussed and reviewed a few more rhythm strips of their patients. Ryan was joyful because finally he is 'getting a hang of' the daunting task of EKG analysis. Jane felt good for mentoring Ryan to be part of the CCU team.

Points to Remember!!!

- Premature atrial contractions are originated and sustained in ectopic pacemakers and abnormal re-entry circuits.
- Premature atrial contraction has a different shaped P wave because of its ectopic origin.
- Occasional PACs are benign; frequent ones are treated with beta-blockers, calcium channel blockers or digoxin.
- Paroxysmal atrial tachycardia by nature has short duration.
- Multifocal atrial tachycardia has different shaped P waves and is also called wandering pacemaker.
- Accelerated atrial rhythms diminish atrial kick.
- Along with nodal blockers, avoidance of stimuli and administration of adenosine or vagal maneuvers are other forms of treatment for paroxysmal atrial tachycardia.
- Multifocal atrial tachycardia is predominantly seen in patients with COPD.
- Antiarrhythmic agents such as flecainide and propafenone are contraindicated in patients with coronary artery disease and left ventricular dysfunction.
- Atrial flutter is produced by re-entry of impulses to the re-entry circuit mostly located on the right atrium.

- Saw tooth waves in atrial flutter are called flutter waves.
- Atrial flutter and fibrillation carry the same risk of having a thromboembolic event and therefore need anticoagulation.
- Rate controlling calcium channel blockers, beta-blockers and digoxin may be helpful in controlling ventricular response in flutter or fibrillation.
- Instead of uniform shape flutter waves, chaotic fibrillatory waves are seen in atrial fibrillation.
- Atrial fibrillation causes loss of atrial contractility, inappropriately fast ventricular response and loss of atrial appendage contractility.
- Risk of having a thromboembolic event in patients with atrial fibrillation can be accessed with CHADS2 scoring system.
- Rate control, prevention of thromboembolic event and rhythm control are basic goals of atrial fibrillation treatment.

Test Your Understanding

1. Which of the following mechanism is responsible for origin of atrial arrhythmia?
A   Impaired contractility
B   Problems with automaticity
C   Impaired conductivity
D   AV node dysfunction

2. The hallmark finding in premature atrial contraction is _____?
A   Presence of multiple P waves between two adjacent QRS
B   Wide and distorted QRS complex
C   Premature PQRST complex
D   Multiple R waves between two P waves

3. Which of the following physiologic mechanism is affected by atrial tachycardia?

A   Loss of contraction of right ventricle

B   Loss of contraction of left ventricular appendage

C   Loss of atrial kick

D   Impaired atrial filling during cardiac cycle

4. Treatment option for paroxysmal atrial tachycardia does not include_____?

A   Adenosine

B   Vagal maneuvers

C   Caffeine ingestion

D   Beta blockers

5. Which of the following statement is not true regarding multifocal atrial tachycardia?

A   It has uniform shaped QRS complex

B   It has uniform shaped P waves

C   There is P waves with different morphology

D   It is commonly seen in COPD

6. Which of the following represent the hallmark symptom of atrial flutter?

A   Bizarre and undulating baseline

B   Chaotic and irregular P waves

C   Presence of uniform shaped flutter waves

D   Atrial contraction above 400 bpm

7. Which of the following statement accurately identifies persistent atrial fibrillation?

A   Episodes that last less than a day

B   Episodes last more than a week

C   Atrial fibrillation lasting less than an hour

D   Episodes lasting a few years

8. Which of the following is not considered as a major risk factor for thromboembolic event in atrial fibrillation?

A   Age greater than 75 years

B   Congestive heart failure

C   Presence of osteoarthritis

D   History of stroke

9. Which of the following is not a treatment option for Afib patients with higher risk of stroke?

A   Use of Coumadin

B   Use of Dabigatran

C   Use of Ibuprofen

D   Use of heparin

10. Which of the following is not a goal of treatment in atrial fibrillation?

A   Control ventricular response

B   Acceleration of atrial response

C   Prevention of blood clots

D   Converting back to sinus rhythm

Answers

1.   B   Problems with automaticity
2.   C   Premature PQRST complex
3.   C   Loss of atrial kick
4.   C   Caffeine ingestion
5.   B   It has uniform shaped P waves
6.   C   Presence of uniform shaped flutter waves
7.   B   Episodes last more than a week
8.   C   Presence of osteoarthritis
9.   C   Use of Ibuprofen
10.   B   Acceleration of atrial response

CHAPTER 7

AV Junctional Rhythms

In this chapter

- Premature junctional contraction
- Junctional bradycardia
- Accelerated junctional rhythm
- Junctional tachycardia
- AV nodal re-entry tachycardia
- Tachycardia with accessory pathways

Clinical scenario

Diane is the intensive care unit RN who was recently moved from surgical ICU to cardiac care unit. She has more than 20 years of experience in medical ICU however, is not familiar with many of the complex heart rhythms. With the new adventure in the coronary care unit, Diane is trying to learn from fellow nurses and physicians. Today she is taking care of Mr. Ramirez, who is a 34 yr old Spanish-speaking gentleman admitted with palpitation and syncope. Diane does not speak any Spanish except few words and therefore was using an interpreter telephone for communicating with Mr. Ramirez. She learned that he doesn't have any past medical history except for occasional 'fluttering' in his chest associated with dizziness for last few years. He works in construction and yesterday evening while at work he had an episode of palpitation and associated dizziness that made him fell off of a small ladder.

Luckily, he landed on the insulation material kept on the floor and sustained no injuries. He denied losing consciousness during this event and felt like 'dizzy and darkness coming to the eyes' right before his fall. According to the report from night shift, patient is admitted to coronary care unit in anticipation for electrophysiology consultation for 'junctional tachycardia'. Around eight o'clock, resident physician from electrophysiology department, Dr. McDowell came to see the patient. After evaluation, Dr. McDowell told Diane that the patient will be going to cath lab for electrophysiology study and possible ablation for AVNRT. Diane, with her limited knowledge about complex heart rhythms was puzzled with the term AVNRT. Willingness to learn from everyone and ability to ask questions without hesitation having the hallmark qualities of her personality, Diane didn't waste a moment and asked Dr. McDowell "I am still learning your jargon in electrophysiology. Can you please explain to me a bit more on this AVNRT? Sorry, I don't have a clue!!". While typing on the keyboard, Dr. McDowell turned around in his chair and said "Yes, of course. I can tell... You know better than anyone here about how to manage HHNK but not AVNRT" Dr. McDowell chuckled. "That's right, at this moment, I can handle HHNK and hepato-renal syndrome much better than any of these complex arrhythmia" Diane replied. "Don't worry, I am just teasing. We are happy to have you at CCU. I am sure your knowledge about hyperglycemic hyperosmolar nonketotic coma and liver failure will be useful for us one day in this unit". McDowell continued "So, in this patient, he developed syncope secondary to tachycardia. If you look at the 12 lead from last night, there were few episodes where patient had dizzy symptoms and palpitation when 12 lead showing AVNRT episodes. But, for your knowledge, let me explain to you some of the basics of junctional tachycardia before we analyze this rhythm".

The junctional rhythm or junctional escape beat is a *pacemaker impulse originating within the atrioventricular node*. As mentioned in the initial chapters, every cardiac cell has the capacity of automaticity, which is the ability to generate its own electrical impulse. AV junction is of no exception. The rate at which the AV node produces impulse is lower than that of the SA node and is about **40 to 60 beats per minute**. Junctional rhythms are usually seen when there are *no electrical impulses coming down from the SA node or anywhere else in the atria*. Since the AV node is sitting in between the atria and the ventricle, electrical impulses originating at the AV node can travel *forward to the ventricles (ante grade conduction)* or *backward up to the atria (retrograde conduction)*.

There are three distinct regions within the AV node that produce electric impulses. They are **high**, **mid** and **low** regions. An Impulse producing at the **high AV node** will travel to the atria first and creates atrial contraction before it produces contraction of the ventricles. The resulting EKG complex will have an **inverted P wave** because of the *backward flow of the* *impulse.* Since the atria are contracting prior to the ventricle, this inverted P wave will be positioned before QRS complex.

In the case of an impulse originating from the **mid** region of AV node, *P wave is usually absent* because it is buried within the QRS complex. In a **low** AV node impulse, electricity spreads to the ventricle before the atria resulting in an inverted *P wave after QRS complex.*

There are three distinct presentations of **P waves** in junctional rhythms such as **inverted, absent** or **trailing**. A short PR interval with any one of the characteristics P wave pattern is the hallmark of junctional rhythm.

Since the AV node is sitting midway between the atria and the ventricle, *PR interval* in these

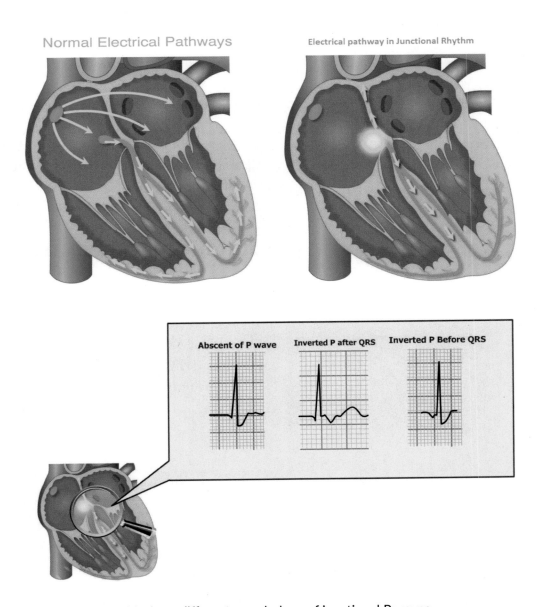

Fig 7.1 Junctional rhythm with three different morphology of junctional P waves

rhythms are *lower than normal* (less than 0.12 seconds). This is because the impulse doesn't take much longer to get from its origin to the AV node, which is represented by PR interval. In nutshell, *a short PR interval with the characteristic inverted, trailing or absent P wave* is the hallmark of junctional rhythm.

Premature Junctional Contraction (PJC)

These rhythms are originating from an *ectopic focus within the AV junction*. Mostly, PJC's are caused by *coronary artery disease, acute myocardial infarction, digitalis toxicity, hypokalemia* or *chronic lung disease*. This beat occurs before a normal sinus rhythm and it depolarizes the *atria retrograde* (backwards) and the *ventricle antegrade* (forward), producing an inverted P wave and a normal QRS complex. As mentioned earlier, depending on the location of impulse origin within the AV node, the P wave can be inverted, absent or trailing.

Basic characteristics are

Rhythm:	underlying regular rhythm, interrupted with the PJC.
Rate:	usually normal.
P wave:	normal except during PJC; inverted, absent or trailing

P wave during ectopic beat.

PR interval:	normal except during PJC where it is *shorter* than 0.12 sec if P wave is present.
QRS complex:	normal.
T wave:	normal, unless P wave superimposes T wave.
QT interval	within normal limits, since ventricular contraction is unaffected.

Clinical significance: most of the time, PJCs are benign and unnoticed. However, in the event either a premature beat produces under filling of the ventricle or it doesn't conduct down the ventricle, patient may feel skipped beat or lightheadedness. *No treatment is needed for asymptomatic PJC.* For hemodynamically significant PJCs, underlying reasons need to be investigated.

Junctional Rhythm

It is also known as the **Junctional escape rhythm** with a heart rate of **40** to **60 bpm** with all the characteristics of junctional type P waves throughout the rhythm. Common causes for junctional rhythms are *increased vagal tone, toxicity with beta and calcium blockers, coronary artery disease, degenerative changes in SA node* etc.

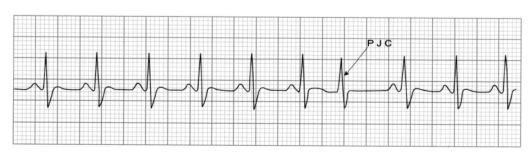

Fig 7.2 Premature junctional contraction

Junctional Bradycardia

The major difference of junctional bradycardia from other junctional rhythms is that, the rate of cardiac contraction will be *less than 40 bpm*. Most of the time, this slow heart rate may result in hemodynamic compromise. Therefore, aggressive management with the use of *transcutaneous* or *intravenous pacemaker* is the treatment of choice for hemodynamically significant junctional bradycardia. *Atropine* may also be useful in this setting.

Accelerated Junctional Rhythm

This rhythm is known as 'accelerated' because it fires impulses *above the inherent rate of junctional tissue*, which is 40 to 60 bpm. Similar to other junctional impulses, they are produced as a **coping mechanism of heart** when the atrial impulses terminate. Along with other characteristics of the junctional rhythm, the rate will be between **60 to 100 bpm**.

Junctional Tachycardia

This type of rhythm happens when an *ectopic junctional focus starts firing at rate above 100 bpm*. This is a form of supraventricular tachycardia where *enhanced automaticity of the AV node* generates fast impulses that essentially suppress the SA node.

Basic characteristics are

Rhythm:	regular
Rate:	*greater than 100*
P wave:	characteristic *inverted, absent or trailing P wave.*
PR interval:	*less than 0.12 second*
QRS complex:	within normal limits
T wave:	normal unless a P wave hides within it.

Clinical significance: retrograde conduction of P wave along with tachycardia can diminish cardiac output. If so, *beta-blockers*, *calcium channel blockers* or *adenosine* maybe the treatment of choice.

"Since you have a basic idea about junctional tachycardia by now, let's see your patient's rhythm", Dr. McDowell said by reaching over to the printer and grabbing the 12 lead EKG printout. "Shelly, can I have a sheet of paper please", Dr. McDowell turned his chair towards the unit secretary and asked. He turned back to Diane

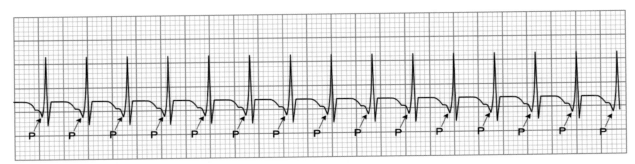

Fig 7.3 Junctional tachycardia

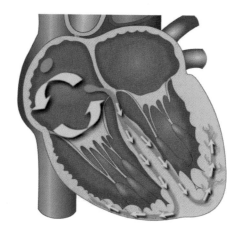

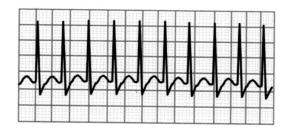

Fig 7.4 AVNRT

with a white paper and said, "Let me draw some pictures first. It is easier to explain the fast and slow pathway if we have a picture on a sheet of paper rather than drawing in thin air". He then started drawing on the paper and continued, "Okay, let's go to the internal mechanism of AV node".

AV Nodal Re-entry Tachycardia (AVNRT)

This is the most common type of paroxysmal supraventricular tachycardia. This rhythm originates because of a peculiar anatomic structure within the AV node. The AV node comprised of myocardial fibers with two distinct depolarization properties. One group has **fast pathway** and *longer refractory time* and the other one has **slow pathway** with *shorter refractory period*. During *normal sinus rhythm, only fast pathway* is manifested in an EKG even though impulses pass through both fast and slow pathways.

A premature atrial contraction (PAC) originating at a critical moment during cardiac cycle will be blocked in the fast pathway because of the longer refractory period. However, a relatively shorter refractory period of slow pathway may allow this impulse to conduct through slow pathway alone. During this slow conduction phase, the fast pathways comes out of their refractory period and therefore available for impulse conduction. The impulse that is conducting through the slow pathway may then get in to the fast pathway circuit and start retrograde conduction, leading to a vicious *re-entry pathway within the AV node.*

The characteristic EKG finding in AVNRT is the *long PR interval of PAC initiating this rhythm,* suggesting *impulse conduction through slow pathway.* Similar to any other junctional rhythm, P waves may either be inverted (retrograde conduction) or absent (buried in T wave).

Basic characteristic are

Rhythm: regular
Rate: *120-250 beats per minute*

P wave: inverted, absent or trailing

PR interval: *longer in the initiating impulse*. Unable to measure if P wave is absent.

QRS complex: narrow and regular

T wave: regular or distorted by buried P wave.

QT interval: normal or varying depending on the T wave.

Clinical significance: In the absence of structural heart disease, AVNRT is usually asymptomatic. However, in presence of coexisting structural heart disease, this rhythm may produce *hypotension* or *syncope*.

Management: Treatment is directed towards altering conduction within AV node by employing *vagal maneuvers*, *adenosine*, *beta-blockers* or *calcium channel blockers*. If the rhythm is refractory to treatment, **synchronous direct current cardioversion** is the treatment of choice. For patients with recurrent AVNRT refractory to medication and cardioversion, **radiofrequency ablation** of slow pathway is an option with high success rate.

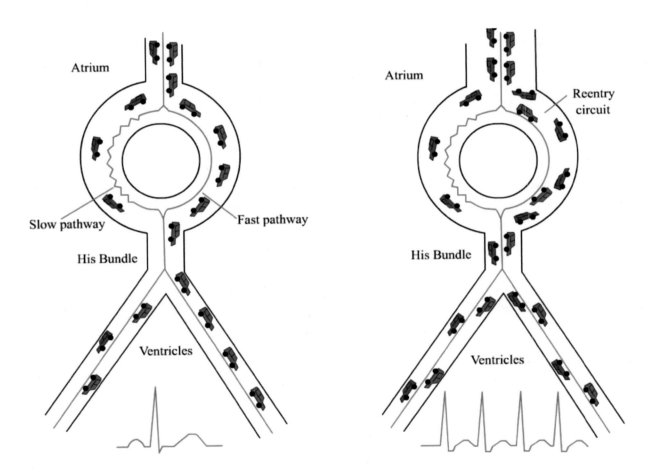

Tachycardia Associated with Accessory Pathways

Fig 7.5 Slow and fast pathway for AVNRT

"So in the case of Mr. Ramirez, are you sure he had AVNRT that caused his syncope episode?" Diane asked. "No, I am not one hundred percent sure. I have asked cardiology to do an echo to see any structural or wall motion abnormalities for him before we proceed with electrophysiology study. Even though he is young and no risk factors for coronary disease, we have to exclude the possibility of underlying structural heart disease", McDowell continued "so keep him starving. I will figure out within next hour which way we are going after talking to my attending. I discussed possible plan of care with the patient and is agreeable". Diane said, "This poor guy is so worried, and he just want to get this resolved so that he can go back to work". "Yeah... we will take care of him", McDonald said by reaching for the binder from the cupboard. Another CCU nurse Tracy, was over hearing the conversation between Diane and Dr. McDowell and asked, "Hey Dr. McDowell, since you have explained this much about reentry tachycardia, can you please clarify one thing for me?" "Yes, of course. Fire away..." McDowell said to Tracy without taking his eyes off of the computer screen he is working on. "I would like to know the difference between AVNRT and WPW. Are they the same?" Tracy asked. McDowell now turned around and looked at Tracy, "Really, you want me to explain that? It is a lame question...." McDowell said while staring at Tracy with a serious face. He quickly changed his expression to a happy face with smile and continued "Just kidding... you know I always joke around you guys". "I know, I know... " Tracy said in a dragged-out voice and continued, "You big guys always joke around....". "No Seriously, I was joking. You know I am always happy to talk to CCU nurses and explain things. I believe this knowledge eventually translate in to better patient care and personally... less headache for me since I don't get calls at the middle of the night because someone is not able to identify the rhythm and what is happening with the patient". "That's true... we have some heart rhythm champions in this unit who can figure out no matter how complex the rhythm is. You know Selma from day shift and Benson from nigh crew?". "I know them very well. As a matter of fact, Ben saved me last week when I was on call because he was able to figure out the rhythm for one of his patient, which was interpreted as aberrancy by the rounding resident when it was a slow V-tach in reality. He called me right away and we were able to take care of it before the patient went in to serious trouble. So, as I said, I really appreciate what you guys are doing". "Good to hear that." Tracy said. "Okay, now back to your question. Both AVNRT and WPW differ fundamentally in the location of reentry circuit. For AVNRT, it is within the right atrium close to the AV node or within the node. The electro physiologic property of these cells are similar to the AV node. For WPW, the pathway exists in the atrioventricular valvular ring and has electrophysiological property of ventricular myocardium. WPW is also known as AVRT or Atrioventricular reciprocating tachycardia. It is bit confusing for beginners. Let me draw a picture for you..." Dr. McDowell paused and then continued. "Uhm,.. I think I have an app in my phone that can show things

much better", McDowell pulled out his phone from his waist pocket and start swiping through it. McDowell showed the three-dimensional picture of the interior of the heart and explained the areas where the abnormal circuits are located and also discussed about the approach they take during ablation procedures. " Wow!! you are a wealth of information. Thank you for your time. I hope we didn't ruin your entire schedule for the day", Tracy said while extending her hand for a shake hand with Dr. McDowell. "You are welcome, as I said, I really appreciate what an amazing job you guys do, so ask me anytime. I am happy to share what I know... As far as schedule for today, I only have two consults so far this morning and all procedures are scheduled for this afternoon. Anyway, Thanks guys. Diane, I will call you once I figure out the plan for your patient". McDowell said by getting up and shaking hands with both Diane and Tracy.

Wolff- Parkinson- White Syndrome (WPW)

Under normal circumstances, an impulse originating from the atria travels down to the ventricle only through the single AV nodal gateway. However, in some situations there is existence of an abnormal connection between the atria and the ventricle called accessory pathway. This short circuit complicates the matter by either *conducting some impulses to the ventricle before AV node does it* or *allowing impulses to enter back to the atria from the ventricle*. In WPW syndrome, this pathway is called Bundle of Kent. WPW is also known as pre-excitation syndrome. This re-entry circuit can create re-entry tachycardia.

When an antegrade conducting accessory pathway exists between the atria and the ventricle, some impulses bypass the AV node through this fast pathway and therefore result in a short PR interval. Since this accessory pathway does not extend throughout the ventricle like the His-Purkinje system, impulse travelling through accessory pathway *cannot initiate a complete ventricular contraction*. So, in the resulting EKG, a characteristic *slurring of initial portion of QRS* known as Delta wave will be present.

In WPW syndrome, the *accessory pathway can act as a re-entry circuit* for the impulse and allows it to return to the atria and can create tachyarrhythmia. The retrograde activation of the atria through accessory pathway is known as echo beat. Compared to the AV nodal pathway, this *accessory bundle serves as a low resistance pathway* for impulse conduction. In patients with underlying atrial fibrillation, because of the low resistant conduction in this accessory channel, fibrillatory waves can travel down to the ventricles bypassing the AV node. This leads to formation of lethal ventricular fibrillation.

Atrioventricular re-entrant tachycardia (AVRT) can have either narrow or wide complex QRS. AVRT with narrow complex tachycardia is called orthodromic AVRT and the one with wide QRS complex as antidromic AVRT. In narrow complex AVRT (Orthodromic), *antegrade conduction is through AV node* and therefore there is *no Delta wave during sinus rhythm*. However, in wide complex AVRT,

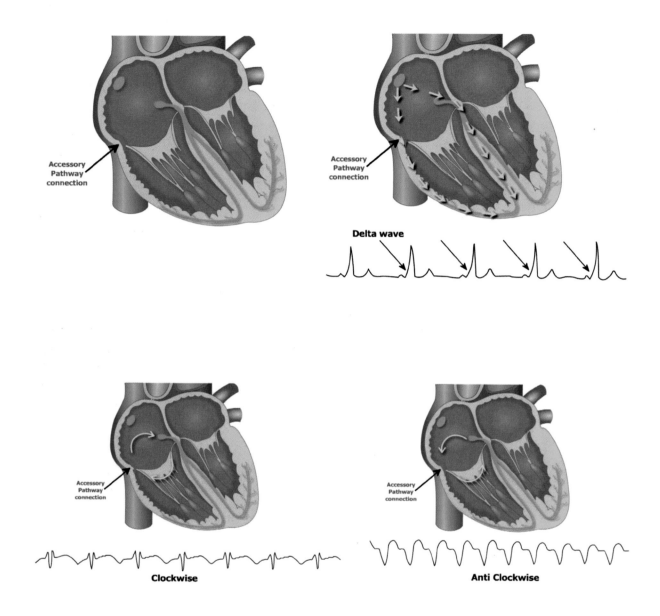

Fig 7.6 **WPW Syndrome (Accessory pathways and possible mechanism of tachycardia)**

forward conduction to the ventricle is through accessory pathway. This create slurred QRS (Delta wave).

Common drugs used for treatment of tachycardia such as beta-blockers, calcium channel blockers or digoxin impart resistance to the AV nodal conduction. If they are used in presence of some AVRT, it may lead to downward conduction of majority of impulses through *path of least resistance*, which is the accessory pathway in this situation. This may produce ventricular tachycardia (V-tach) or fibrillation (V-Fib).

Therefore, *it is very important to identify presence of Delta wave before treating tachycardia.*

Atrial fibrillation with WPW can create a wide QRS complex tachycardia resembling V-tach. The major differentiation between ventricular tachycardia and atrial fibrillation with WPW is that *ventricular tachycardia is usually regular; however, latter is irregular.* WPW syndrome is associated with congenital anomalies such as Ebstein anomaly, mitral valve prolapse and hypertrophic cardiomyopathy (HCM). These patients generally have AV nodal re-entry tachycardia, atrial fibrillation or flutter.

Asymptomatic patients with WPW do not need any treatment. Definite management of WPW is a radiofrequency catheter ablation of the re-entry pathway and is the primary treatment of choice if possible. Depending on the type of AVRT, *intravenous beta-blockers* or *Procainamide* can be useful for suppression of tachycardia in acute phase. Procainamide is of special importance because of its ability to depress conduction and prolong refractoriness except that of the AV node. For patients with infrequent episodes of AVRT, *Propafenone* and *Flecainide* can be used in long-term.

Ashman's Phenomenon

This is a form of aberrant conduction commonly associated with Atrial fibrillation. A premature atrial impulse form after a long RR interval will be conducted aberrantly (through an alternate pathway within the ventricle) because one bundle branch is not completely recovered from the previous impulse. In general, Right bundle has a slower refractory period than that of Left bundle and therefore the *resulting impulse has a Right bundle branch block configuration* of **rsR'** pattern. It usually results in a small number of wide complex beats on an otherwise narrow complex rhythm.

There is so called Long Short rule for Ashman Phenomenon as follows. *The earlier in the cycle the PAC occurs and the longer the previous cycle, more likely the PAC will be conducted through aberrant pathway within the ventricle.* Clinical significance of Ashman' phenomena is that it should be differentiated from serious preexcitation conditions such as WPW syndrome.

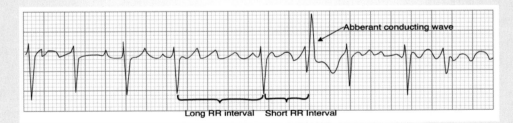

Fig 7.7 Aberrant conduction with Ashman's phenomenon

Box 7.1 **Ashman's phenomenon**

Clinical scenario

During the course of the day, Diane's patient was seen by Cardiology team and evaluated for structural heart disease. In the afternoon, he went for electrophysiology study and came back after successful ablation of AVNRT. With a great deal of new knowledge, Diane was able to give a detailed shift endorsement to the night crew. The night shift RN was very much impressed with Diane's advanced knowledge of complex heart rhythms.

Points to Remember!!!

- Junctional rhythms originate within the atrioventricular node and are characterized by inverted or absent or trailing P waves and a short PR interval.
- Rate of junctional impulse is between 40 to 60 beats per minute.
- Common causes of junctional rhythms are increased vagal tone, drug toxicity, degeneration of SA node and coronary artery disease.
- Accelerated junctional rhythm is a junctional rhythm with heart rate greater than 60 beats per minute.
- Junctional tachycardia has rate of greater than 100bpm.
- AV nodal re-entry tachycardia (AVNRT) is the most common type of paroxysmal supraventricular tachycardia.
- Characteristic EKG finding in AVNRT is the long PR interval in PAC, which initiate this arrhythmia because of involvement of the slow conduction pathway in the AV node.
- AV nodal blocking agents, vagal maneuvers, DC cardioversion or radiofrequency ablation of the slow pathway are the possible treatment options for AVNRT.

- WPW syndrome is caused by abnormal conduction through accessory pathway known as bundle of Kent.
- WPW is also called pre-excitation syndrome because of the activation of ventricle through accessory pathway before the AV node.
- Premature activation of ventricles through accessory pathway cause formation of slurred QRS complexes called Delta waves.
- In certain situations like in atrial fibrillation, the accessory pathway acts as a low resistance pathway for downgrade moment of impulses and can cause ventricular fibrillation.
- Narrow complex QRS tachycardia in atrio ventricular re-entrant tachycardia (AVRT) is called orthodromic AVRT and one with wide complex called antidromic AVRT.
- It is important to identify presence of accessory pathways before treating re-entry tachycardia, because of the possibility of causing ventricular fibrillation by blocking AV node and facilitate conduction through accessory circuit.
- Radiofrequency ablation is a definite and most desired treatment option for atrio ventricular re-entry tachycardia.

- Procainamide and intravenous beta-blockers are preferred treatment for acute management of re-entrant tachycardia.
- Propafenone and flecainide can be used for prevention of infrequent AVRT.

Test Your Understanding

1. Which of the following is not a characteristic of junctional rhythm?

A   Heart rate in 60 to 80bpm
B   Inverted P wave
C   Short PR interval
D   Heart rate in 40 to 60 bpm

2. Junctional rhythm may be caused by _____?

A   Decreased vagal activity
B   Increased vagal tone
C   Use of atropine
D   Discontinuation of beta-blockers

3. Which of the following represent the heart rate of accelerated junctional rhythm?

A   20 to 40 bpm
B   40 to 60 bpm
C   60 to100 bpm
D   Above 100 bpm

4. Which of the following pathway is actively involved during normal AV nodal conduction?

A   Slow pathway with long refractory period
B   Fast pathway with shorter refractory period
C   Fast pathway with long refractory period
D   Short pathway with shorter refractory period

5. Treatment for AVNRT does not include_____?

A   Vagal maneuvers
B   Adenosine
C   Atropine
D   Beta-blockers

6. Which of the following represents the accessory pathway of WPW syndrome?

A   Bundle of His
B   Thorel's tract
C   Bundle of Kent
D   Buckman's pathway

7. WPW syndrome EKG is characterized by_____?

A   J point elevation
B   Delta wave
C   Multiple P waves
D   Inverted T waves

8. Which of the following is the most desirable treatment option for WPW syndrome?

A   Amiodarone
B   Oral beta-blockers
C   Radiofrequency ablation
D   Use of Flecainide

Answers

1.   A   Heart rate in 60 to 80bpm
2.   B   Increased vagal tone
3.   C   60 to 100 bpm
4.   C   Fast pathway with long refractory period
5.   C   Atropine
6.   C   Bundle of Kent
7.   B   Delta wave
8.   C   Radiofrequency ablation

CHAPTER 8

Atrio Ventricular Block

In this chapter

- First-degree heart block
- Second-degree type I heart block (Wenckebach)
- Second-degree Type II heart block (Mobitz type II)
- Third degree AV block

Clinical scenario

'Get me the crash cart', CCU RN Dave yelled at Rick who is the new CCU RN under training. Rick was on his way back from lunch and was expecting to meet CCU educator Martha at the nurse's station so that he can go over with her on the training schedule. Rick ran to the corner and pushed the cart towards the room where Dave was standing. When he arrived, Rick saw the patient is still sitting in the recliner with his head leaning over the over bed table. Dave was shaking on his shoulder and asking, "Are you okay Mr. Simpson?'. The patient replied in a low tone of voice "I am dizzy, feeling very week". "Rick, get me the external pads from the defibrillator. This guy is in third degree", Dave said to Rick. By the time rick grabbed the external pads from the pouch atop the defibrillator, three more nurses rushed in to the room. " Sorry Dave, we were at a code blue in room 20. That's why it took so long", Gloria, who is the member of CCU rapid response team said with a heavy sigh and continued "So what is happening, I see him in third degree with rate of 28". "Yes, he

was admitted with anterior MI and is supposed to go for angiogram this afternoon. He was in first degree till now and suddenly progressed in to third" Dave said while placing the defibrillator electrodes on the chest and back of the patient with help of Rick. Jeremiah, who is another rapid response team member quickly connected the defibrillator to the patches and said "Okay, I am going to start pacing him at seventy, alright". "Yah, go ahead", Dave said while looking at the monitor and continued. "Guys, we have capture at seventy. Can any one page Dr. Branson from cardiology please. He is supposed to take the patient to cath lab this afternoon. He may have to take him sooner than that". After few minutes of externally pacing Mr. Simpson, he felt good. Blood pressure stabilized, and patient is no longer symptomatic. Dave had started the patient on low dose Dopamine and the patient was taken to cath lab within ten minutes. After all the events, Rick met with his unit Educator. Dave had already told her how quick Rick responded to his call and helped him to take care of the patient during emergency. Both Dave and Martha congratulated him for such a prompt response. Dave said, "Martha, we need to train this guy well. He got good skills for a CCU RN and also is a good team player. He will be an asset to the unit". "I think so too", Martha said while tapping to Rick's shoulder. After few minutes of discussion about their schedule, Martha told Rick, "So today, since you had an incident with a patient in heart block, let's review the topic of various types of heart block".

In normal conduction system of the heart, impulses originating from the SA node spread across the atria and channels down to the AV node. At the AV node, these impulses are delayed due to so-called **decremental conduction** and thereby allowing atrial depolarization. Hence, the AV junction serves as the *natural regulator* or *signal point* of ventricular response with its inherent delaying mechanism. However, during atrioventricular block this *delaying mechanism becomes so profound* that either the *delay at the AV junction increases* or some of the atrial beats *does not conduct* down to the ventricle.

There are varying degrees of heart blocks identified. The site of block can be either in the AV node itself or sometimes at the bundle branches. In this chapter, we will discuss about the heart block involving AV node. Varying degrees of bundle branch blocks are discussed later in 12 lead EKG interpretation session. Depending on the severity of the AV block, it can be **first-degree heart block**, **second-degree type I** (Wenckebach), **second-degree Type II** (Mobitz type II) and **third-degree heart block** (AV dissociation).

First-Degree Heart Block

More than usual delay in conduction through the AV node creates the hallmark EKG change in first-degree heart block as *elongated PR interval*. Even though an increased delay exists, all

Heart Block

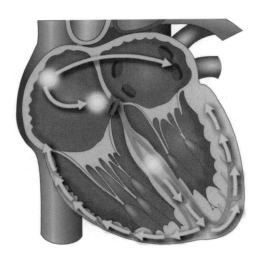

Fig 8.1 **Heart block**

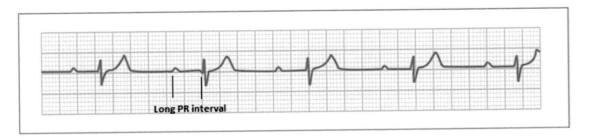

Fig 8.2 **First-degree heart block EKG (Note the presence of long PR interval)**

the impulses get through AV node and complete its conduction.

Basic characteristics are

Rhythm: regular
Rate: both atrial and ventricular rates within normal limits.
P wave: normal and uniform. One P wave for each QRS complex.
PR interval: *greater than 0.2 second*.

QRS complex: normal and uniform.
T wave: within normal limits.
QT interval: unaffected.
Clinical significance: First-degree heart block *by itself is benign*. It is usually caused by *coronary artery disease* causing *AV nodal ischemia*, medications like *beta-blockers*, *calcium channel blockers* and *digoxin* etc. Treatment of underlying causative factor is the management strategy.

Second-Degree Type I Heart Block (Wenckebach)

In this type of heart block, there is a *periodic conduction failure* within the AV node causing *PR interval to progressively lengthen until a drop in QRS complex*. After this dropped beat, the cycle repeats forming groups of beats called **footprint of Wenckebach**. Unlike first-degree heart block, *all the atrial beats do not conduct to ventricle* during Wenckebach phenomena.

Basic characteristics are

Rhythm:	regularly irregular, especially at dropped QRS.
Rate:	atrial rate 60 to 100; ventricular rate varies with degree of block.
P wave:	normal and uniform.
PR interval:	*varies from beat to beat with a progressive lengthening, until a complete drop of QRS.*
QRS complex:	normal and uniform except during missed beats.
T wave:	normal and is absent in missed QRS.
QT interval:	not measurable during missed beat.

Clinical significance: second-degree type I heart block has the *same causative factors as first-degree heart block*. Mostly patients are asymptomatic. However, for symptomatic patients they may need *transcutaneous* or *transvenous pacing*. This rhythm has a small chance of progressing into more serious type of heart blocks and therefore requires close observation.

Second-Degree Type II Heart Block (Mobitz Type II)

This type of heart block is more serious than Wenckebach. In these patients, the location of block can either be at the AV node or at the bundle branch. Characteristic EKG shows *a regular rhythm with constant PR interval from beat to beat until a* **sudden drop of complete QRS complex**. There is a high likeliness that this *rhythm can progress to the third-degree heart block* and therefore needs immediate attention. Most of the patients have coexisting bundle branch blocks with a wide QRS complex. Occasionally, the block can be seen in regular pattern such as 2:1 or 3:1 conduction, where the QRS drops after every two or after every three P waves respectively.

Basic characteristics are

Rhythm:	regular atrial rhythm and irregular ventricular rhythm.
Rate:	atrial rate usually within normal limits; however, ventricular rate is lower than the atria.

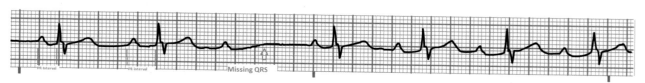

Fig 8.3 Second degree type I Heart block

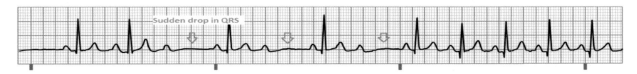

Fig 8.4 Mobitz type II

P wave: normal and uniform.

PR interval: unable to determine at missed beats.

QRS complex: normal and uniform except in missed beats and wide if a bundle branch block present.

T wave: normal size and configuration except in missed beats.

QT interval: not measurable during missed beats.

Clinical significance: If left untreated, this rhythm can progress into *serious AV dissociation*. Mobitz type II heart block is usually caused by *hypoxia*, *myocardial infarction*, *conduction system disturbance* etc. Depending on the extent of block in these patients, it may cause significant reduction in cardiac output. Symptomatic bradycardia with concomitant conduction block may respond better with *epinephrine than atropine*. Transvenous or transcutaneous pacing is the other available option for immediate treatment with transition to permanent pacemaker implantation depending on the reversibility of underlying causes.

Clinical scenario

"Does this second-degree heart block always prelude third degree?", Rick asked Martha. "No, not necessarily. As you see in the patient this morning, sometimes third-degree heart block starts without warning. It depends on the underlying pathology. Remember, there is redundancy built in the heart for pacemaker function. If a higher order pacemaker fails to activate in time, an ectopic focus downstream will take over the function. But, if there is extensive damage in conduction between the chambers, both chambers will start firing their own impulses and is what happening in third degree. Let's look at the patient's EKG", Martha said and then grabbed Mr. Simpson's chart and turned tabs for EKG tab. "Yes, this is the one from this morning. let's look at it together". Martha said Rick and pushed the chart towards him.

Third Degree AV Block (AV Dissociation)

This is the most serious type of heart block. In natural conduction system of the heart, the atria contract first and send blood down to the ventricles and then the ventricles contract. This ensures optimal cardiac output. During third-degree heart block, there is no electrical connection between upper and lower chambers

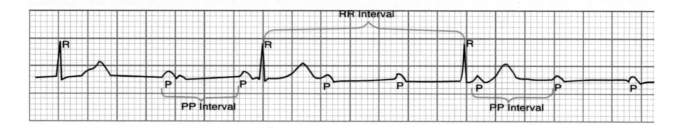

Fig 8.5 Third degree heart block

and therefore there is no synchronized contraction. Here, atrium fires impulses from the SA node at its own rate and contract accordingly. At the same time, since there is no electrical impulse from upper part of the conduction system, an ectopic focus within the ventricle start generating escape rhythm. This eventually leads to *atrial contraction at one rate* and *ventricular contraction at a different rate*. Since there is no synchronization between these chamber contractions, serious hemodynamic compromise can occur immediately.

Basic characteristics are

Rhythm:	grossly irregular; however, regular atrial and ventricular rhythms.
P wave:	regular and uniform; however, not associated with QRS complexes. *P-P interval is constant.* Sometimes it gets buried in to QRS or T wave.
PR interval:	not measurable and there *is no corresponding QRS for each P wave.*
QRS complex:	regular and uniform. Narrow or wide morphology depends on presence of bundle branch block. *R-R interval constant.*

T wave: normal and uniform.

Clinical significance: AV dissociation cause significant hemodynamic compromise and therefore patients are usually symptomatic. Third degree heart block is usually caused by the same causative factors as in Mobitz type II heart block. *Transcutaneous* or *transvenous pacing* is a definite choice for immediate treatment. These patients may need permanent pacemaker implantation for long term unless the causes are reversible.

Clinical scenario

"So, now you know a great deal about heart block, isn't it?" Martha asked Rick. "Yes, I do, your explanations provide me a clear understanding of what to look for in identifying the heart block. As a matter of fact, I was quite impressed with Dave and Gloria when they were able to instantly recognize the rhythm and swing in to action. They seem to be very experienced and knowledgeable in heart rhythm". "You will be too..." Martha said with a smile and continued "It takes some time for anyone to instantly recognize these rhythms. But with practice, you also will be able to do it. Now,

let's go and ask Dave about that patient from this morning", Martha got up. Both Rick and Martha went to Dave and asked about the patient. Dave told them that the patient had angioplasty with stent placement to proximal Left anterior descending coronary artery. He is going for second part of his angioplasty to Right coronary artery in next 48 hours. Now the patient has a transvenous temporary pacemaker inserted through the left femoral vein and is being paced by temporary external pacemaker. Martha and Dave discussed with Rick about the temporary pacemaker and showed him how to connect it and how to change the settings if needed. At the end of the day, Rick was happy that not only he was involved in saving life of a critically ill patient, but also was able to learn important topics with hands on experience.

Points to Remember!!!

- First-degree heart block is characterized by an elongated PR interval than normal because of a delay in conduction at the AV node.
- Causative factors for the first-degree heart block are AV nodal ischemia and toxicity from AV nodal blocking agents.
- In second-degree type I (Wenckebach) heart block, there is progressive prolongation of PR interval until a drop in QRS complex.
- In second-degree Type II (Mobitz type II) there is a sudden drop in QRS complex with no warning signs.
- Second-degree Type II heart block needs urgent attention because of its tendency to progress into third degree heart block.
- In third degree heart block, atrio ventricular contraction is asynchronous.
- In third degree heart block, P-P and R-R interval are constant; however, there is no association between occurrence of P and R waves.
- Immediate transcutaneous or transvenous pacing with advancement to permanent pacemaker implantation is the mode of treatment for third degree heart block.

Test Your Understanding

1. Which of the following statement is true for second-degree type I heart block?

A   Constant PR interval throughout the rhythm

B   Constant PR interval until a drop in QRS complex

C   Progressive lengthening of PR interval until a complete drop in QRS

D   Elongated QT interval throughout the rhythm

2. Which of the following represents the value of PR interval in first-degree heart block?

A   0.15 second

B   0.12 second

C   0.19 seconds

D   0.24 seconds

3. Which of the following is not accurate for second-degree Type II heart block?

A   QT interval may be constant from beat to beat

B   There is one P wave for every QRS complex

C   There is complete PQRST complex missing intermittently

D   QRS complex are missed intermittently

4. Which of the following is the most detrimental effect of third degree heart block?

A   Absence of atrial contraction

B   Absence of ventricular contraction

C   Formation of blood clots

D   Atrioventricular dissociation

5. Treatment options for third degree heart block include_____?

A   Digoxin

B   Amiodarone

C   Transcutaneous pacing

D   Defibrillation

Answers

1.   C   Progressive lengthening of PR interval until a complete drop in QRS

2.   D   0.24 seconds

3.   C   There is complete PQRST complex missing intermittently

4.   D   Atrioventricular dissociation

5.   C   Transcutaneous pacing

CHAPTER 9

Ventricular Rhythms

In this chapter

- Premature ventricular contraction (PVC)
- Idioventricular rhythm
- Agonal rhythm
- Accelerated Idioventricular rhythm
- Ventricular tachycardia
- Torsade's de Pointes
- Long/short QT syndrome
- Ventricular fibrillation
- Asystole

Clinical scenario

Harry is the emergency room RN precepting student nurse Martin in the busy Memorial Care hospital ER. Even though it is only nine o clock in the morning, they already had two STEMI runs and few critically ill patients. Now, Harry and Martin are attending Mr. Kalinowski, a 69-Year-old male patient with a heavy accent, admitted for epigastric pain that started last night. He was cracking jokes with Martin and Harry about how his thick Polish accent got him in trouble when he first came to United States 40 years ago. Harry was establishing IV lines and Martin was asking health history questions. Mrs. Kalinowski was at bedside. 'How's it going?'. Martin turned around when he felt the hand on his shoulder. It is Dr. Paul, the ER physician on duty, passing by Mr. Kalinowski's bed. "It's going good". Martin replied. Harry, while trying to prepare the IV site looked at Dr. Paul and said "We can't complain. If we do, there's no time for anything else". Harry chuckled. Dr. Paul who is an ex-marine, smiled and walked away saying "Aye, Aye Captain". Harry went on with inserting the IV and was ready to leave the bedside. All of a sudden, Harry heard Mr. Kalinowski snoring. When he looked up, the patient appears to have eyes rolled to the top. The bedside monitor start alarming. Both Martin and Mrs. Kalinowski were distracted at this time. Bedside monitor showed wide complex heart rhythm at the rate of 160 bpm. Harry put his hand on Mr. Kalinowski's shoulder and shook him and asked, "Hello Sir, are you ok?" There was no response from the patient. Harry quickly reached over the head of the bed and pushed code blue alarm and started chest compression after a brief assessment of carotid pulse. In a matter of seconds, the ER code team sprang into action and started providing advanced cardiac life support measures. The patient was eventually defibrillated and intubated. He was taken to cardiac catheterization lab for emergency coronary angiogram as the EKG post resuscitation showed changes suggesting ST elevation myocardial infarction involving anterior wall of the heart.

An hour later, Martin and Harry got to sit together in the staff hub for morning break and rehashed the events happened with this patient. Martin asked, "what just happened?". Harry smiled and replied "my friend, welcome to the real life in ER. Things can go bad in a matter of moment in this place. The guy passed out with ventricular tachycardia, that probably might have been an indication of sudden cardiac ischemia from ST elevation MI". While opening a can of soda, Harry continued "it is very typical picture in the emergency room. This patient presented with epigastric pain, that must have been unstable angina and a myocardial infarction in the making for last few hours. All of a sudden, a rapid change in coronary blood flow possibly from a plaque rupture and acute closure of the artery caused ventricular tachycardia. This form of tachycardia will not produce a rhythm that provides cerebral perfusion. The guy passed out and what we heard was sudden snoring". "Wow, that was intense" Martin replied while biting off a chunk from the burrito he had in his hand.

Ventricular rhythms are originated from an ectopic focus within the ventricle. Since the propagation of this impulse to the myocardium and resulting ventricular depolarization are sluggish compared to its normal counterpart, these rhythms generate *wide and bizarre QRS complexes* with duration more than 0.12 seconds. Because of the fact that it originates in the ventricle, most of these impulses don't have an atrial component and some of them have retrograde conduction to atria. Some of this retrograde conduction from ventricular beats combined with antegrade SA node conduction creates fusion beats. Fusion beats can be distinguished from other PVCs because, *it happens at the exact timing as a normal SA nodal beat* supposed to occur and has *different shape* compared to other PVCs.

Because of the disorganized ventricular depolarization, the *T wave usually assumes opposite direction of the QRS complex* during ventricular rhythms. Even if the atrial component is present, resulting P wave will be buried within the wide QRS complex. Because of the lack of effective atrial contraction and disorganized ventricular depolarization, these rhythms may not provide adequate cardiac output.

Ventricular pacemaker cells have an inherent pacing rate of 20 to 40 bpm. However, during certain situations they can produce ventricular rate up to 200 bpm because of the presence of re-entry circuits. These tachyarrhythmias produce *no effective cardiac output* and therefore are detrimental to the person's life.

Premature Ventricular Contraction (PVC)

Premature ventricular contractions are ectopic beats originate within the ventricle and are mostly benign in nature. They may originate from a single ectopic focus in the ventricle or from multiple foci. If they originate from a single focus, they are uniform in appearance (unifocal). Waves with varying morphology (Multifocal) are seen in rhythms originating from multiple foci. They are either isolated or at times occur at regular intervals such as every other beat (bigeminy) or every third beat (trigeminy). They may also come in pairs known as couplets. If there are *more than three beats in a row*, it is termed as a run of VT. Since the retrograde conduction of ventricular impulse can cancel out atrial stimuli coming down through the AV node, mostly there is complete or incomplete compensatory pause following PVCs. This represents the time taken by the SA node to regain its function.

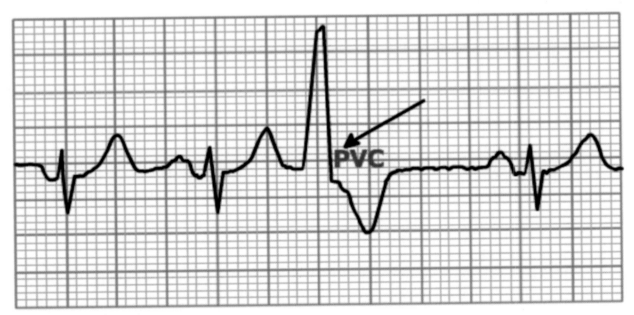

Fig 9.1 Premature ventricular contraction

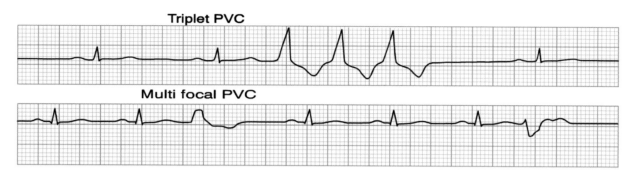

Fig 9.2 Various forms of Premature Ventricular Contractions (PVC)

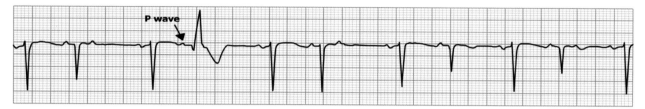

Fig 9.3 PAC with aberrant conduction (Note the p wave before distorted QRS).

Premature atrial contraction (PAC) with aberrant conduction may also produce wide and bizarre QRS complex. This aberrant rhythm should be distinguished from that of ventricular tachycardia. *Presence of a premature P wave at the beginning of tachyarrhythmia* or *typical right or left bundle branch block pattern of QRS complex* are the tell-tale signs of differentiating **PAC with aberrant conduction** from that of **Ventricular tachycardia (V-tach)**. Therefore, it is important to see the origin and termination of tachyarrhythmia to differentiate true versus aberrant rhythms.

Basic characteristics are

Rhythm:	underlying regular rhythm with irregularity during PVC.
Rate:	usually within normal limits.
P wave:	normal except during PVC, where it is absent.
PR interval:	normal except during PVC, where it is immeasurable.

QRS complex:	*wide and bizarre duration >0.12 second during PVC.*
T wave:	*points in opposite direction of QRS deflection* (if QRS negative, T wave positive).
QT interval:	not measurable during PVC.

Clinical significance: Premature ventricular contractions are common among *old age* and patients with *structural heart disease*. They are also seen in *electrolyte imbalance, acidosis, congestive heart failure, acute myocardial infarction, drug toxicity* etc. Occasional PVCs are benign. However, if they occur more frequent especially in the setting of underlying structural heart disease, they can progress to lethal ventricular tachycardia or fibrillation.

If the PVC originate in the **down slope of T wave** of the previous repolarization wave, it can produce **polymorphic ventricular tachycardia (R on T phenomena or Torsades de Pointes).** *Magnesium deficiency* is one of the common condition precipitate this arrhythmia.

Management: Treatment of underlying pathology like *correction of electrolytes (potassium, magnesium)* is of supreme priority during treatment of symptomatic PVCs. Anti-arrhythmic agents like *Amiodarone* and *beta-blockers* may be helpful in frequent PVCs. Recurrence of multiple PVCs in high frequency can create a reversible cardiomyopathy that can further impair ventricular function. It is important to remember when using anti arrhythmic drugs that many of these drugs themselves can create ventricular arrhythmias (pro arrhythmic effect) by slowing down conduction in the ventricles (Q-T prolongation). Therefore, judicious use and adequate monitoring is needed while treating patients with these medications to prevent sudden cardiac death (SCD) from lethal arrhythmia.

Idioventricular Rhythm

This is a true ventricular rhythm with a rate of 20 to 40 bpm and is a tell-tale sign of *imminent life-threatening events* like *agonal rhythm* or *asystole*. This is also known as ventricular escape rhythm. It usually happens when all the higher-level pacemakers have failed. Mostly, this rhythm does not provide sufficient left ventricular contraction and leads to serious hemodynamic compromise. At times, this rhythm accompanies *complete AV dissociation* (third degree heart block).

Basic characteristics are

Rhythm:	regular.
Rate:	*20 to 40 bpm*.
P wave:	none except in third degree heart block.
PR interval:	immeasurable.
QRS complex:	wide and bizarre with greater than 0.12 seconds duration.
T wave:	like PVC, deflects in opposite direction of QRS.
QT interval:	prolonged.

Clinical significance: This rhythm *may or may not produce a pulse*. Hence, these individuals require aggressive management with *basic and advanced cardiac life support* measures.

Accelerated Idioventricular Rhythm (AIVR)

Accelerated Idioventricular rhythm originates due to *abnormal automaticity* within the ventricle. This rhythm produce impulse at 40 to 120 bpm. It can be seen in the absence of any structural heart disease or in the event of *acute myocardial infarction*, *cocaine toxicity*, *digoxin intoxication*, *postoperative cardiac surgery* or after *chemical or mechanical*

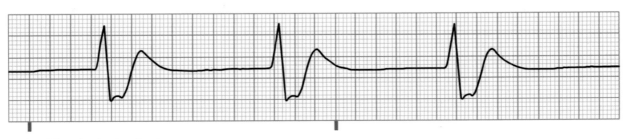

Fig 9.4 Idioventricular rhythm

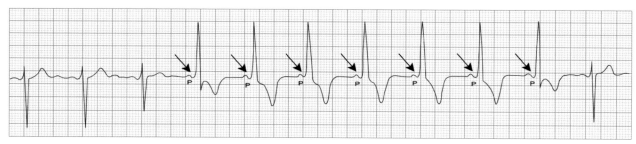

Fig 9.5 AIVR (Note the presence of P waves and brief self-limiting pattern of arrhythmia)

revascularization of coronary arteries as in **tPA administration** and **coronary angioplasty**. In these settings, it is also known as **reperfusion arrhythmia**.

The basic characteristics that differentiate **AIVR** from that of **slow** V-tach are its *gradual onset and termination with a brief self-limiting pattern*. In order to differentiate **Idioventricular rhythm (IVR)** from **accelerated Idioventricular rhythm (AIVR)**, *look for presence of P waves in AIVR that is absent in Idioventricular escape rhythm*. Remember *in AIVR, SA node is still firing unlike in IVR* where there is no higher order pacemaker functioning.

AIVR does not produce significant compromise in cardiac output in many instances as the ventricles are contracting at a decent rate. In the setting of acute myocardial infarction or post-operative status, sustained AIVR may produce hemodynamic instability due to lack of AV synchronization.

Basic characteristics are

Rhythm:	mostly regular.
Rate:	*40 to 120 bpm.*
P wave:	may be seen *before, during* or *after QRS*. At times, *inverted* or *absent*.
PR interval:	immeasurable if P waves are absent.
QRS complex:	*wide and bizarre*, duration >.12 seconds.

QT interval: prolonged.

Clinical significance: As mentioned earlier, hemodynamic compromise rarely occurs with AIVR. Mostly it is a self-limiting arrhythmia.

Ventricular Tachycardia

Ventricular tachycardia (V-tach/ VT) forms when there are *three or more PVCs in a row* and *ventricular rate exceeds 100 bpm*. If the duration of ventricular tachycardia is less than 30 seconds, it is called **non-sustained ventricular tachycardia (NSVT)**. If the rhythm *persists for more than 30 seconds* or terminated within 30 seconds by either an Automated Implantable Defibrillator (**ICD** or **AICD**) or external defibrillation, it is known as **sustained VT**. Depending on the morphologic characteristics, VT can be classified into **monomorphic VT** and **polymorphic VT**.

Basic characteristics are

Rhythm:	usually regular.
Rate:	*ventricular rate between 100 to 250 bpm*; atrial rhythm is indiscernible.
P wave:	usually absent or indistinguishable.
PR interval:	not applicable.
QRS complex:	*wide and bizarre* with the duration >0.12 seconds.

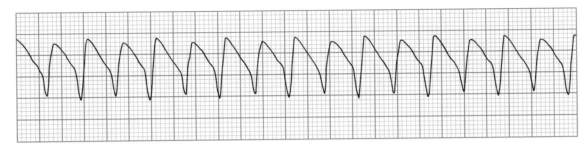

Fig 9.6 Monomorphic VT

T wave: in the opposite direction of QRS deflection.

QT interval: prolonged.

Clinical significance: Depending on the duration and frequency of ventricular tachycardia, it may be well tolerable or having serious hemodynamic effects. *Cardiac output is considerably reduced* with contraction of ventricles at 150 to 250 bpm as it *does not provide time for effective ventricular contraction.*

Management: Any VT or V-Fib that is compromising hemodynamic function should be treated with immediate **asynchronous DC cardioversion** if available. Intravenous **Lidocaine** or **Amiodarone** are other mainstay treatment choices. *Intravenous antiarrhythmics should be continued even after electrical cardioversion* in order to prevent recurrence of these rhythms. *Basic and advanced cardiac life support* is indicated if the patient doesn't have a perfusing rhythm.

Evaluation of wide complex tachycardia is extremely important as there are some entities that resemble ventricular tachycardia, but not in as lethal as VT. Some of these rhythms are **pacemakers mediated wide complex tachycardia** and **SVT with aberrancy**. Most important characteristics that differentiate ventricular tachycardia from other nonlethal wide complex tachycardia are

1. A wide complex QRS that *does not match previous* wide complex tachycardia.
2. Absence of any pre-excited QRS pattern in sinus rhythm *at the beginning* of wide complex tachycardia.
3. The *bizarre QRS pattern that does not mimic right or left bundle branch block* in a 12 lead EKG.
4. *Slurring of initial part of QRS.*
5. *Signs of AV dissociation in the EKG like fusion beats.*

Unlike wide complex supraventricular tachycardia, *VT does not respond to vagal measures* or other standard treatment for SVT. In majority of situations, ventricular tachycardia is seen in patients with prior cardiac structural damage that is evident in EKG by presence of Q waves.

Clinical scenario

Heather and Jenny are working in the critical care unit. Heather is a seasoned critical care nurse and Jenny is a nursing student who is in critical care rotation. They had a busy day, packed with one code blue and another patient who had to go Cath lab for ST changes in EKG following angioplasty.

Finally, both got to sit together and talk about their day. Sitting in the corner cubicle in front of the computer, Heather asked. "I know the day was action-packed and I don't know how much you were able to comprehend from what all things happened around us today. Do you have any particular questions?" By flipping the pages of her pocket note pad, Jenny replied. "I wanted to talk to you about both patients. Let me ask about the first one who had code blue. In the beginning of the code blue, I heard someone saying it is torsade's. What was that?" Heather turned around in her chair towards Jenny and replied. "Torsades is a form of ventricular tachycardia. It is also called polymorphic ventricular tachycardia. In this rhythm, the QRS complexes was up and down in an undulating fashion. Let me see whether the monitor captured the rhythm. Let's go to the telemetry station". Heather and Jenny got up and walked towards telemetry station. Heather pulled out the patient's alarm history and scrolled through recorded alarms around the time of the code blue. "It was around 11:30, right? "Heather asked. Jenny nodded her head and said, "I think so, because it is right before I was planning to go to lunch". "Here it is", Heather replied by clicking the rhythm strip on the touchscreen monitor. "Look here". Heather continued. "See this rhythm, all these waveforms are going up and down. These up-and-down waveforms are actually QRS complexes. You can see these waveforms progressively get bigger and bigger to a point where the biggest waveform and then start coming down in their amplitude. You can also see the pattern is repeating. This is very typical for Torsades. The problem with this rhythm is that it can go to Vfib if not treated". "Yeah, I see what you're saying. It's almost like waxing and waning in its amplitude". Jenny said, pointing her finger to the enlarged rhythm strip in the monitor.

Torsades de Pointes (TDP)

This is the form of polymorphic ventricular tachycardia with a *varying QRS morphology*. It has an *undulating QRS complex* with reference to the isoelectric line. This rhythm can degenerate into ventricular fibrillation with serious hemodynamic compromise. The French term *Torsades de Pointes* means 'twisting of the points'. This rhythm may be produced by conditions like acute *ischemia* or myocarditis and is generally not a reproducible rhythm like monomorphic VT during an electrophysiologic evaluation. Since TDP refers to a more serious unstable situation, urgent treatment is warranted.

Basic characteristics are

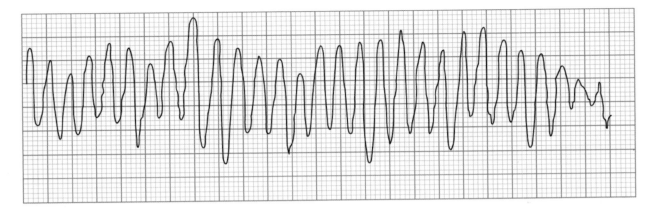

Fig 9.7 Torsades (Polymorphic VT)

Rhythm: may be regular or irregular with varying QRS size.

Rate: atrial rate immeasurable, *ventricular rate 150 to 300 bpm.*

P wave: not seen.

PR interval: unable to calculate.

QRS complex: *wide and bizarre* with the duration greater than *0.12 seconds.* Complexes with *positive and negative deflection* are present compared to isoelectric line.

T wave: difficult to identify.

QT interval: prolonged in beats prior to Torsades.

Clinical significance: Torsades is considered as one of the lethal arrhythmias since it can degrade into ventricular fibrillation with serious hemodynamic compromise. *Short runs of Torsades are generally well tolerated* in the absence of critical hemodynamic issues. If longer, it is *treated with the same measures* as of *sustained ventricular tachycardia.*

Management: Hallmark treatment for Torsades is intravenous administration of **magnesium** since *hypomagnesemia at myocardial level* can precipitate this rhythm. Same as that of VT, *Torsades can be produced by pharmacologic agents* like *Procainamide* and *Amiodarone,* which are known for their Q-T prolongation property (**pro-arrhythmic effect**). Therefore, frequent monitoring of QT interval is warranted, especially in the beginning of treatment with these medications.

VT Storm

Repeated ventricular tachycardia episodes requiring electrical cardioversion or defibrillation with *more than two incidents within 24 hours* are defined as **VT storm**. In reality, these patients experience much more episodes than stated in the definition. In the absence of long QT interval prior to the VT episode, active **myocardial ischemia** or fulminant **myocarditis** should be suspected.

Management strategy differs depending on whether the VT is polymorphic or monomorphic in nature. In patients with recurrent monomorphic VT, intravenous administration of *Amiodarone, Lidocaine* and *Procainamide* may prevent recurrence. However, these QT prolonging drugs can make the patient arrhythmogenic because of their proarrhythmic property. Radiofrequency ablation of foci within the ventricle is of great use in *refractory VT*. In the case of polymorphic VT, possible management options include correction of electrolyte imbalance like magnesium and potassium, stopping any Q-T prolongation drugs, treatment of underlying myocardial ischemia etc.

Other Forms of Ventricular Tachycardia

Long QT Syndrome (LQTS)

This is a *congenital defect in cardiac ion channels* responsible for repolarization of myocardium. In the action potential curve of myocardial tissue, this defect enhances *sodium and calcium inward movement* and *inhibits outgoing potassium ions* during **phase 1** (plateau phase). It essentially prolongs action potential duration *and therefore QT interval*. When the QT is abnormally prolonged, there is more chance for possible ectopic beats to produce polymorphic VT events (R on T phenomena or Torsades). This is especially significant during exercise or activity where QT interval is short in proportion with increase in heart rate.

Most patients with long QT syndrome, *corrected QT interval* is up to 460 ms *in men and* 480 ms *in women*. Q-T prolongation beyond 500 ms suggests higher risk for arrhythmia. QT prolonging drugs like Sotalol can precipitate long QT syndrome in individuals who are otherwise asymptomatic. Therefore, close monitoring is warranted during initiation of these drugs. For patients with prolonged QT interval greater than 500 milliseconds and those with strong family history of sudden cardiac death (SCD), implantation of an Implantable Cardioverter Defibrillator (ICD) is the treatment of choice for primary prevention of SCD.

Short QT Syndrome (SQTS)

This is one of the relatively uncommon syndromes with effective QT interval less than 320 ms with EKG finding of tall T waves. These patients are more prone to have *fibrillation of atria or ventricle*. These patients require Implantable cardioverter defibrillator (ICD) implantation to prevent sudden cardiac death from V-Fib. In certain situations, because of the presence of tall T waves, ICD may count them as QRS complex (effectively doubling the number of

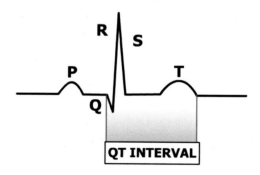

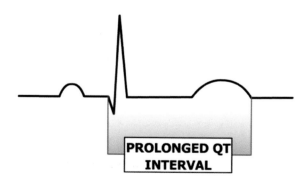

Fig 9.8 Long QT syndrome

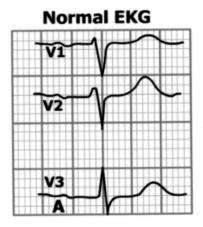

Normal EKG — V1, V2, V3 (A)

Brugada syndrome — V1, V2, V3 (B)

Fig 9.9 Brugada pattern (Note the characteristic ST segment elevation in V1-V3

calculated QRS complexes) and inappropriately Institute shock therapy for tachyarrhythmia.

Brugada Syndrome

Brugada syndrome was named after Spanish cardiologists who identified this genetic disorder as the reason for many unexplained sudden cardiac deaths in Southeast Asian males. This involves mutation of SCN5A gene that *reduces inward sodium movement* during **phase 0** of action potential in myocardial cells located at the epicardium of the right ventricular outflow tract. This leads to dramatic shortening of cardiac action potential of these cells compared to the rest of the ventricle. Therefore, these cells may undergo abnormal repolarization and depolarization circuits compared to the rest of the myocardium, resulting in lethal ventricular arrhythmia. Patients with Brugada syndrome has EKG showing complete or incomplete **right bundle branch block pattern** with characteristic **coved-type** (In lead V2 as shown in Fig 9.10) or **saddle back** (as in lead V3 in Fig 9.10) ST elevation in V1 to V3 in sinus rhythm.

These patients require *ICD implantation* as they are at high risk of having lethal ventricular

arrhythmia leading to sudden cardiac death. The *family members should be screened* for presence of this disorder. Misdiagnosis of ventricular tachycardia resulting from Brugada syndrome and subsequent treatment with class I antiarrhythmic drugs (sodium channel blocking agents like Procainamide and flecainide) may exacerbate chances of lethal arrhythmia.

Major Drugs Causing QT Prolongation

Drug	Use
Amiodarone	Antiarrhythmic
Chloroquine	Antimalarial
Chlorpromazine (Thorazine)	Antipsychotic
Clarithromycin	Antibiotic
Erythromycin	Antibiotic
Disopyramidine (Norpace)	Antiarrhythmic
Dofetilide (Tykosin)	Antiarrhythmic
Droperidol	Anti-nausea
Methadone	Opiate agonist
Procainamide	Antiarrhythmic
Sotalol (Betapace)	Antiarrhythmic
Quinidine	Antiarrhythmic
Thioridazine	Antipsychotic

Box 9.1 Major QT prolonging drugs

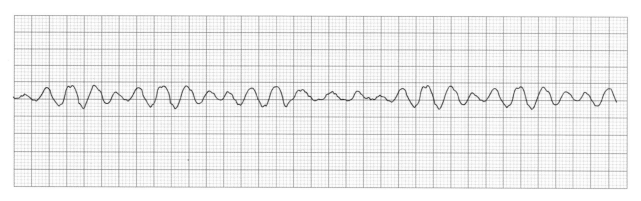

Fig 9.10 **Corse V Fib**

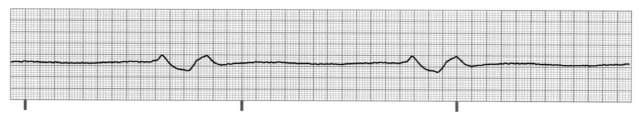

Fig 9.11 **Agonal rhythm**

Ventricular Fibrillation (V Fib)

V fib is a *completely disorganized and chaotic ventricular rhythm* with serious hemodynamic implications. Multiple ectopic foci within the ventricle start firing impulses, leading to unsystematic depolarization of the ventricles. Resultant 'quivering' motion of ventricles produces **ventricular standstill**. V fib can be with coarse or *fine fibrillatory waves*.

Basic characteristics are

Rhythm:	*completely irregular, with fibrillatory waves.*
Rate:	cannot be determined.
P wave:	not seen.
PR interval:	cannot calculate.
QRS complex:	no definite QRS; *just undulating waves.*
T wave:	not seen.
QT interval:	cannot calculate.

Clinical significance: Causative factors are the same as that of ventricular tachycardia however, indicate more serious underlying events. This rhythm does not generate any cardiac output whatsoever. Therefore, immediate basic and advanced life support measures including **emergent defibrillation** is a necessity. If left untreated, coarse V fib may progress to fine V fib. Pharmacologic agents such as *Amiodarone* and *Lidocaine* are used after electrical defibrillation to prevent recurrence of VT/V fib.

Osborn wave

These waves are otherwise known as hypothermia waves where there is a *positive deflection seen at the J point* (Junction between QRS complex and ST segment). They are more prominent in the precordial leads. This is a characteristic EKG finding in patients with either accidental or therapeutic hypothermia.

These waves usually *resolve with rewarming of the patient*. These waveforms should be differentiated from that of Brugada syndrome or early repolarization. Even though controversy still exists, Osborn waves are considered as a *warning sign of ventricular fibrillation* in hypothermic patients.

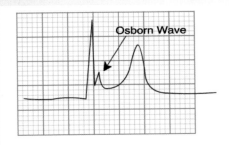

Fig 9.3 C Osborn waves

Box 9.2 Osborn waves of hypothermia

Agonal Rhythm

Agonal rhythm is the *worst possible cardiac rhythm second to asystole*. It denotes severely impaired cardiac function with impending death. Even the ventricular escape beats are not produced enough to maintain an Idioventricular rhythm. Characterized by irregular occasional wide complex beats.

Basic characteristics are

Rhythm: irregular.
Rate: *less than 20 beats per minute.*
P wave: none.

PR interval: not applicable.
QRS complex: wide and bizarre with greater than 0.12 seconds duration.
T wave: swing in opposite direction of QRS.
QT interval: prolonged.

Clinical significance: As mentioned earlier, agonal rhythm is the last possible electrical impulses before asystole. *Severe and massive cardiac compromise* has already happened. The patient may essentially be in shock state. Management of underlying reversible causes or aggressive life support measures with *basic and advanced cardiac life support* is the treatment of choice.

Sally is a student nurse working with John at the step-down unit. Out of the 3 patients, one of them was a 93-year-old female with pancreatic cancer. The patient was in Do Not Resuscitate (DNR) code status. This patient was steadily deteriorating from the beginning of the shift and finally passed away around noon. John and Sally worked together to prepare the body for morgue. Both of them came back and sat for lunch together and talked about the patient. "Are you turned off by today's patient's death?" John asked, "I see you don't seems to be happy". "Yes I am, this is the first time I am seeing anybody dying. I just don't feel right about it. It almost feels like sick to my stomach when trying to eat my lunch" Sally said by putting her left hand on her forehead. "It's okay, I know it can be hard in the beginning. Most of us went through these phases. But think about it, death was the best solution for that patient? She's a 93-year-old lady with pancreatic cancer, which one of the worst. She never looked like someone who can survive extensive treatment or surgeries. Actually, I'm glad that you had such an experience during your student life. It helps you to understand the spectrum of things we as nurses involve on a daily basis. We have to be prepared as a nurse to care for patients at all phases of life including death. Now, I think there are many things that you might have observed for that patient. Let me point this one out for you. Did you notice the rhythm all this morning for that patient?" John asked. "Yes, I did. But it was so overwhelming for me that I didn't get a chance to ask you" Sally said while trying to retrieve a spoon from her lunch bag and continued. "I never saw such rhythm for any other patient". "It was something called agonal rhythm" John said. He continued by sipping from a can of soda "it is very slow, like heart rate of around 20 or 30 per minute with a weird wide complex rhythm. I'll show you when we get back to the nurses' station after lunch. This rhythm was actually followed by a flat line when she finally passed away. It is called asystole or complete standstill of the heart". "Oh, that makes sense now what I was seeing in the telemetry. You know what, I don't think I can eat." Sally said by putting the bowl of yogurt and spoon back to the lunchbox. "I need some time. This is too much for me. I am going to go for a walk and will be back in 15 minutes" Sally said after getting up from the chair. "I can see, first time it can be very disturbing to watch somebody dying. It's okay to take some time to get out of it, but I don't recommend skipping your lunch" John said with a smile. He continued "take your time. Maybe it is worth talking to your educator and some of your fellow students about this to get their perspective. Don't worry about the time. Just go and talk to them. It is worth sharing the experience and talk about it so that you all can reflect and learn from it. I will talk to your clinical educator when she comes around. Are you okay going by yourself, if not I'll walk with you". "I'm okay, I just need some time. Yes, I'm going to talk to my classmates and educator. I will be back, thank you." Sally said and walked out of the staff hub.

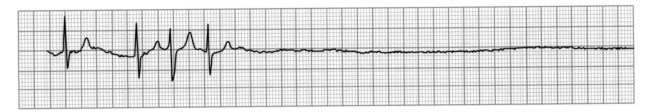

Fig 9.12 Asystole

Asystole

This denotes a *complete ventricular standstill* with no cardiac output. In the EKG, a flat line appears, and it essentially means there is absolutely no pacemaker activity anywhere in the heart. In some instances, we may see some atrial activity with no corresponding ventricular response. If the patient has a pacemaker either permanent or temporary, we may see pacing spikes at regular intervals without corresponding P or QRS complex.

Basic characteristics are

Rhythm: atrial-irregular if present, ventricular-none.
Rate: indiscernible.
P wave: may or may not be present.
PR interval: not measurable.
QRS complex: not present.
T wave: not seen.
QT interval: not applicable.

Clinical significance: This is the terminal rhythm of the heart. Usually seen after *profound cardiac damage* in severe *hypoxia, multisystem failure* etc. Aggressive resuscitative efforts with *epinephrine, atropine* and *CPR* are the way to go. If this rhythm persists even after reasonable efforts, it is time to declare demise of the patient.

Points to Remember!!!

- Premature ventricular contractions produce rhythms with wide and bizarre QRS complexes having duration more than 0.12 sec.
- In PVC's, T wave follows the opposite direction of that of QRS complex because of the disorganized ventricular repolarization.
- Ventricular pacemaker cells have an inherent pacing rate of 20 to 40 bpm.
- PVC is can be unifocal or multifocal depending on the ectopic focus and its morphology.
- In terms of regularity, PVCs can be every other beat (bigeminy), every third beat (trigeminy) or more than three in a row called 'run of VT'.
- PACs with aberrancy can be distinguished from PVCs by the presence of premature P wave at the beginning of tachyarrhythmia.
- PACs are common in old age, patients with structural heart disease or in electrolyte imbalance.
- Antiarrhythmic agents like Amiodarone, beta-blockers and correction of underlying causative factors are the modes of treatment for PVCs.

- Idioventricular rhythm or ventricular escape beat with a rate of 20 to 40 bpm is a sign of life-threatening events of the heart.
- Agonal rhythm with a rate less than 20 beats per minute shows massive impairment of cardiac function.
- Accelerated Idioventricular rhythm with the heart rate of 40-120 beats per minute is caused by abnormal automaticity within the ventricle.
- AIVR is considered as a reperfusion arrhythmia in the event of revascularization procedures.
- The main differentiating factor between Idioventricular rhythm (IVR) and accelerated Idioventricular rhythm (AIVR) is the presence of P waves in AIVR.
- If the duration of ventricular tachycardia is less than 30 seconds and terminated spontaneously, it is called non-sustained ventricular tachycardia.
- If the VT episode lasts more than 30 seconds or is terminated within 30 seconds by defibrillation, it is called sustained V-tach.
- VT can be monomorphic and polymorphic depending on the morphology of QRS complex.
- Ventricular tachycardia does not provide any significant cardiac output and therefore immediate intervention is demanded for sustained ventricular tachycardia.
- Asynchronous DC cardioversion for rhythm conversion and use of Amiodarone and Lidocaine for prevention of recurrent is the mode of treatment for ventricular tachycardia.
- Torsades the Pointes can produce ventricular fibrillation and serious hemodynamic dysfunction.
- Hypomagnesaemia is the most common causative factor for TDP.
- Incidence of more than two ventricular tachycardia episodes within 24 hours requiring electrical cardioversion or defibrillation is known as VT storm.
- Radiofrequency ablation of the focus within the ventricle is the treatment for VT storm.
- Long QT syndrome is caused by congenital defect in cardiac ion channels causing prolongation of phase 1 in action potential curve; leading to prolonged QT.
- Corrected QT interval above 500 ms suggests higher risk of arrhythmia in patients with long QT syndrome.
- Implantation of ICD for prevention of sudden cardiac death is the treatment option for long QT syndrome.
- Short QT syndrome with QT interval less than 320 ms can cause atrial or ventricular fibrillation.
- Brugada syndrome is a genetic disorder, common in Southeast Asian males causing sudden cardiac death.
- Characteristic EKG finding in Brugada syndrome is the right bundle branch block pattern with ST elevation in V1 to V3.
- The family members should be screened for presence of gene mutation that can cause Brugada syndrome in patients with this disorder.
- In ventricular fibrillation, disorganized and chaotic ventricular rhythm leads to ventricular standstill.

- Emergent defibrillation is the treatment options for ventricular fibrillation.
- Asystole is the terminal rhythm of the heart that requires aggressive resuscitative effort with CPR and advanced cardiac life support.

Test Your Understanding

1. Which of the following QRS complex duration represent possible ventricular rhythm?
A   0. 0.8 seconds
B   0.04 second
C   0.14 second
D   0.7 seconds

2. Treatment option for frequent PVCs include_____?
A   Atropine
B   Lisinopril
C   Amiodarone
D   Epinephrine

3. Which of the following is true statement regarding Idioventricular rhythm?
A   It is caused by abnormal automaticity within the ventricle
B   It is of no significant clinical value.
C   It shows imminent life-threatening events
D   It has distinct P wave in front of every QRS complex

4. Which of the following possible rhythm can be seen after administration of thrombolytic medications in an acute myocardial infarction patient?
A   Sinus arrhythmia
B   Atrial fibrillation
C   Accelerated Idioventricular rhythm

D   Idioventricular rhythm

5. Sustained ventricular tachycardia is defined as _____?
A   Self terminated within 30 seconds
B   Require defibrillation or last more than 30 seconds
C   Last less than 30 seconds but doesn't require defibrillation
D   Last less than 30 seconds and rate stays within 100bpm

6. What is the most important differentiating factor between Torsades de Pointes and other forms of monomorphic ventricular tachycardia?
A   Presence of wood wide and bizarre QRS complex
B   Ventricular rate 100 to 250 bpm
C   Long QT interval
D   QRS complex with positive and negative deflection

7. Identify the most important electrolyte under consideration in a patient with polymorphic ventricular tachycardia?
A   Calcium
B   Sodium
C   Potassium
D   Magnesium

8. Which of the following is the most desirable treatment for VT storm?
A   Beta-blockers
B   Calcium channel blockers
C   Radiofrequency ablation
D   Digoxin

9. Untreated long QT syndrome may lead to _____?
A   Sinus tachycardia
B   Atrial fibrillation

C   Polymorphic VT

D   Asystole

10. Which of the following statement is true regarding Brugada syndrome?

A   It is caused by intake of large amounts of mercury

B   It involves genetic mutations that alter ionic movement in cardiac cells

C   It involves genetic mutations that change position of the heart

D   There is no evidence for Brugada syndrome to run in the family

11. What is the most common characteristic of Brugada syndrome pattern?

A   Left bundle branch block pattern

B   ST elevation in V5 and V6

C   ST depression in V1 to V3

D   Right bundle branch block pattern with ST elevation in V1 to V3

12. Which of the following treatment option is ideal for the patient in ventricular fibrillation?

A   Cardiopulmonary resuscitation

B   Synchronized cardioversion

C   Emergency defibrillation

D   IV calcium administration

13. Which of the following statement is true regarding hemodynamics during coarse ventricular fibrillation?

A   Coarse V-Fib does not require defibrillation as in the case of fine V-Fib

B   Coarse V-Fib does not cause complete ventricular standstill

C   Courses V-Fib cause physiologic standstill for cardiac output

D   In coarse V-Fib, distinct P waves are easily identified

14. Which of the following EKG parameter has to be monitored while starting a patient on Sotalol?

A   Shortened QT interval

B   Atrial flutter

C   Prolonged QT

D   Short runs of SVT

Answers

1.   C   0.14 second
2.   C   Amiodarone
3.   C   It shows imminent life-threatening events
4.   C   Accelerated Idioventricular rhythm
5.   B   Require defibrillation or last more than 30 seconds
6.   D   QRS complex with positive and negative deflection
7.   D   Magnesium
8.   C   Radiofrequency ablation
9.   C   Polymorphic VT
10. B   It involves genetic mutations that alters ionic movement in cardiac cells
11. D   Right bundle branch block pattern with ST elevation in V1 to V3
12. C   Emergency defibrillation
13. C   Courses V-Fib cause physiologic standstill for cardiac output
14. C   Prolonged QT

CHAPTER 10

Cardiac Electrical Assistive Devices

In this chapter
- Classification of pacemakers
- Modes of pacing
- Paced rhythm
- Complications of pacemaker therapy

Clinical
scenario

Scott is a new respiratory therapist student doing clinical rotations in intensive care unit. He is working with his preceptor Isabel, who is a veteran respiratory therapist in the unit. Both of them participated in the code blue on telemetry floor this morning and came back to ICU for continuing their work. When preparing ventilator and other settings for upcoming cardiac surgery patient in the surgical ICU, Isabel asked Scott about his experience with the code blue. "It was very interesting experience for me", Scott said. "For the first time, I was able to see things in action other than in our simulation lab how a code blue scenario rolls out. I just have one question", Scott continued. "I did not understand why the patient needed a pacemaker placed by the ICU physician who was managing the code". "Good question", Isabel responded. "Did you see the patient became bradycardic while they were trying to resuscitate?" Isabel asked. "Yes, I did and then they were trying to give her atropine, right?" Scott asked. "Yes, but the patient was still bradycardic even after the resuscitation and so they decided to put a temporary pacemaker", Isabel replied while trying to connect the oxygen flow meter to the wall outlet. "So what is the difference between a permanent and a temporary pacemaker?" Scott asked. "You know what, I'll get you to the best person who can answer these questions for you. Let's go and see whether Jackie is available. She is one of the expert nurses in this unit, who can tell you all about this. Let's go over there", Isabel said. Both Isabel and Scott walked over to the nurses' station where Jackie was sitting in front of a computer. "Hey Jackie, this young man has some questions about pacemakers. I thought I'll bring him to the right person to ask. Can you help him please?" Isabel asked. "Absolutely, my pleasure", Jackie turned around and replied. And she continued "what exactly you want to know?" "Oh sorry, this is Scott. I didn't introduce him to you. I apologize", Isabel said. "That's okay, I saw him a few times this morning running after you. I figured he is working with you today". Jackie said. Then she continued, "okay Scott, now what exactly you want to know about pacemaker?". "We were attending a code blue this morning, and the physician put in a temporary pacemaker. I don't know anything about pacemakers. So, I was trying to find out why only a temporary pacemaker not a permanent?" Scott asked. "Oh, you're talking about the code blue in six south this morning, right? I was there too", Jackie replied. "That patient was bradycardic after we resuscitated her from cardiac arrest. In these emergency situations, patient may require electrical stimulation support through a pacemaker temporarily. She may or may not need a pacemaker for long-term. If she requires one, they'll put one in electively", Jackie said. "So, there is permanent and temporary pacemaker?" Scott asked. "Yes, there are different classifications for pacemakers depending on the duration of use, how many chambers are being paced, how the pacemaker is behaving and so forth. You know, in simple terms pacemaker is a programmable computer. Its job is to provide electric impulses to the heart when its natural pacemaker fails", Jackie replied. Then she continued, "we generally use temporary pacemakers in the intensive care unit. They are placed through one of the bigger veins like femoral or internal jugular to the right ventricle. For temporary pacemakers, the pacemaker generator is an external unit that usually sits at the bedside. Let me show you one. Come with me", Jackie got up and walked towards the supply room. Both Jackie and Scott went to the supply room. Jackie opened one of the cupboards and pulled out a small black bag. She opened the bag and took out the temporary pacemaker unit. "See this, this is a unit that connects to the end of the pacemaker lead that we put in the right ventricle. Here are the positive and negative terminals. This is a cable that connect between this unit and the end of the leads comes out of the patient", Jackie said by pointing to the pacemaker cable in the packet. "Now, this is the actual pacemaker lead that the physician will place through a venous sheath", Jackie continued by showing the unopened pacemaker lead. "See these two terminals, this is where the end of this pacemaker cable connects", Jackie explained. Then she continued, "now, for the permanent pacemaker unit, there is no big box like this temporary pacemaker. It is usually the size of a dollar coin or slightly bigger and is placed in a muscle pocket under the collar bone. That is usually done in the Cath Lab. I think Bob has a patient going for pacemaker today. If you're around when the patient comes back, I'll show you how that incision looks like", Jackie said. "Oh, that would be great. I appreciate your help. Thank you for telling me all these. I'll try to read about pacemakers tonight", Scott replied. "Not a problem, happy to help. Please let me know anything else I can help you. It is fun to share the knowledge", Jackie said when walking back to the nurse's station.

Modern pacemakers are technological marvels that provide electrical impulses when the natural pacing or conducting properties within the heart fails. They are indicated for patients with various disorders of automaticity and conductivity. There are various classifications of pacemakers based on their function, duration of use and number of chamber paced.

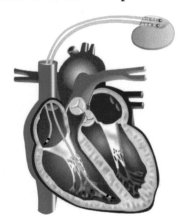

Fig 10.1 Dual chamber Pacemaker

Classification of Pacemakers

Based on the functional significance, pacemakers can be divided into **Fixed** pacemakers and **Demand** pacemakers.

Fixed pacemakers are the old generation of pacemakers with minimal programming options. Here, the pacemaker fires impulses to the designated chamber at a *fixed rate irrespective of the patient's innate cardiac activity*. In normal human beings, this mod of pacing is dangerous as the pacemaker can pace at inappropriately faster rates. This pacing mode may also initiate impulses at inappropriate timing within the cardiac cycle (e.g. on the downslope of T wave) and generate dangerous arrhythmia. This limited functionality provide limited use for this type of pacemakers in the real world.

On the other hand, **Demand pacemakers** are devices that generate impulses *based on the person's innate cardiac impulse*. These types of devices have a preset range of programming (usually 60-120 bpm) and the device *will pace only when the person's heart rate drops below or above the set rate*. These devices make more sense in the real world since they can support the heart when it is in **demand**.

Another classification is based on the number of chambers being paced. It can be

1. **single chamber** pacemaker, which is *either sensing or pacing the atrium or the ventricle*

2. **dual chamber** with *pacing and sensing function in the atria and the ventricle.*

For patients with SA node dysfunction where there is deficiency in impulse production, an **atrial pacemaker** is helpful by providing much-needed electrical stimuli in the atria. This impulse will then carry through normal conduction pathways down to the ventricle and generate cardiac contraction. For patients with conduction defect such as *complete heart block, single chamber pacemaker does not work* because of the *lack of atrio-ventricular connection.* In this instance, sensing the atria and pacing ventricle in synchronized fashion will improve hemodynamics. Essentially, one of the basic concepts of dual chamber pacemaker is to provide **atrio-ventricular synchronization.**

There is a new generation of devices called **biventricular pacemakers**, which are particularly useful in patients with *depressed ventricular ejection fraction* with *coexisting bundle branch block.* Instead of *contracting together,* both ventricles *depolarize in sequence* due to the delay in impulse conduction from bundle branch block. Because of this, whichever ventricle contracts first may partially push the inter-ventricular septum into the adjacent ventricle and therefore losing part of its contractile effort to pump blood out through aorta and pulmonary artery.

Cardiac Resynchronization Therapy (CRT) using biventricular pacemakers ensure *simultaneous contraction of both ventricles.* Many of these patients have underlying structural heart disease with severely reduced ventricular ejection fraction. They require Implantable cardioverter defibrillator (ICD) for

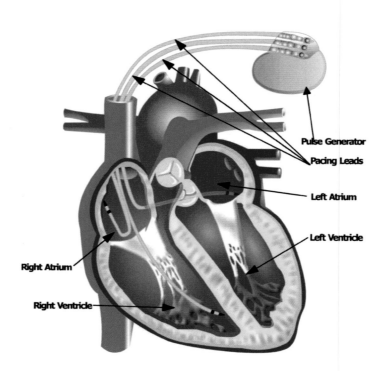

Fig 10.2 Biventricular pacemaker

prevention of sudden cardiac death (SCD). A combined biventricular ICD (BiV ICD) is of common use in this situation. This device has both *pacemaker and defibrillator function for possible ventricular tachyarrhythmia emergencies*. In a BiV ICD, left ventricular lead is placed in the coronary sinus as the pacemaker leads are not generally placed in the left ventricle. Coronary sinus is situated on the roof of the left ventricle and therefore provides indirect access to left ventricular wall.

Depending on the duration of use, pacemakers can be permanent **pacemakers** or temporary pacemakers.

Temporary pacemakers are usually inserted through femoral or jugular veins and are intended for short-term use while the patients are being stabilized. Most common reasons for temporary pacemaker insertion are *fulminant inferior wall myocardial infarction*, *post cardiac surgery*, *third degree AV block* etc. There is increased chance for complications like *infection*, *bleeding* and *lead displacement* with this type of pacemakers. As soon as the patient is stabilized, these devices are either removed or changed for a permanent pacemaker. Alternate access sites for temporary pacing are transcutaneous (with large pads attached to skin), epicardial (during and immediately post cardiac surgery) and transthoracic (by insertion of a needle into the right ventricle and threading pacemaker wire in to the heart) route.

Permanent pacemakers are indicated for long-term use with extremely long battery life (average 5-8 years). They consist of pacemaker leads that are implanted commonly through right or left subclavian vein into the myocardium. There can be up to 3 leads depending on the type of pacemaker. The other ends of these leads are connected to the pacemaker generator

unit that generally implanted in the infraclavicular fossa (underneath the clavicle). These devices can be programmed externally with the use of specialized magnetic probes and therefore are more convenient and user friendly in the real world.

Indications for pacemakers

- Sinus bradycardia (rate less than 40 bpm with pauses)

- Complete atrio-ventricular block (third degree heart block)

- Symptomatic second-degree AV block

- Exercise induced second-degree or third-degree block

- Significant vasovagal symptoms

- Second-degree Type II AV block with wide QRS

- Idioventricular rhythm

Box 10.1 Indications for pacemakers

Modes of Pacing

Modern pacemakers can be programmed in such a way that they provide most individualistic treatment protocol for the given patient depending on underlying disease process. There are mainly five letters used to denote specific programming of the pacemaker. They are mentioned in Box 10.2 with details. Sometimes, only first three letters are used since these represent majority of the pacemaker's capabilities.

Let's look through some examples of pacemaker programming. For the sake of explanation, we are considering only first four letters

Modes of Pacing

First letter	Chamber paced
V	Ventricle
A	Atria
D	Dual or both
O	None .
Second letter	**Chamber sensed**
V	Ventricle
A	Atria
D	Dual (Atria and Ventricle)
O	None
Third letter	**Pacemaker response to intrinsic rhythm**
T	Triggered (trigger pacing in response to a sensed event)
I	Inhibit (inhibits pacing in response to a sensed event)
D	Dual (It can inhibit and trigger impulses in various chambers depending on the event)
O	None(It does not respond to the sensed event)
Forth letter	**Rate response**
R	Rate responsive (pacemaker provide paced impulse for a pre-determined range of heart rate)
O	No rate response
Fifth letter	**Pacemaker's response to tachyarrhythmia**
P	Override pacing for tachycardia available
S	Shock therapy (available in high-energy devices e.g. AICD)
D	Dual-ability to pace and shock
O	None

Box 10.2 Modes of pacing

since the fifth letter is exclusively for high-energy devices like ICD.

VVIR Pacemaker

The first letter **V** stands for chamber paced i.e. *ventricle*. Second letter **V** denote the chamber sensed and, in this example, it is *ventricle*. Third letter **I** shows the response of pacemaker to the patient's own rhythm and here it is *inhibition*. That means, if the pacemaker sees patient's own ventricular beat, it doesn't produce pacemaker impulse. The last letter **R** corresponds to *rate responsiveness* of this pacemaker, which is explained later in this chapter. In nutshell, a **VVIR** pacemaker is functioning as a *single chamber pacemaker with pacing and sensing of ventricle. It does not generate an impulse if the patient has his own ventricular beat.*

DDDR Pacemaker

The pacemaker has ability to pace *both chambers* (first letter **D**- dual), ability to sense from *both chambers* (second letter **D**- dual), ability to inhibit and trigger in *different chambers* (third letter **D**- dual) and has *rate responsiveness* (fourth letter **R**- rate response). In a patient with **DDDR** pacer settings, the device will *look for intrinsic impulse in both chambers*. If there is no atrial impulse, pacemaker will fire at the atria and thereby generate atrial contraction. If the patient has impulse from his own SA node, the pacemaker inhibits its firing since there is no need for an additional impulse.

Coming to the ventricles, the same response happens with pacing from device. If the patient has his own ventricular beat, the devise does not generate a ventricular impulse. Otherwise the device will wait for a pre-determined timeframe (in milliseconds) to see whether the atrial impulse is creating a ventricular response (remember, *AV nodal delay*) before making decisions of how to respond.

This explanation can create some confusion regarding the sequence of pacemaker activity in relation to the letters we mentioned earlier. However, it is important to remember that the device is constantly sensing the cardiac activity and taking decisions within microseconds to create an appropriate response for individual beats of the heart. The pacemaker has inbuilt **programmed timeframe** in milliseconds for which the device will wait before initiating either pacing or inhibition.

Rate Responsiveness

In order to better understand the significance of rate responsiveness along with other programming options, let's take the example of a patient with atrial fibrillation who has a DDDR pacemaker. As mentioned earlier, one of the basic ideas of a dual chamber pacemaker is to *provide AV synchronization*. In this situation, the atrial lead sense *multiple P waves,* usually in the order of 350 to 700 beats per minute because of atrial fibrillation. Due to the innate nature of AV node, most of these impulses get blocked at the AV junction and the patient will have a controlled ventricular response, which produce decent hemodynamics.

In presence of a pacemaker, if the pacemaker was trying to track each P wave in the atria and to generate corresponding QRS complex within the ventricle, this patient will have extremely fast and dangerous ventricular response. In order to prevent this from happening, the rate response mechanism is activated. This provides a range of atrial beats (60-100 in this situation) under which the pacemaker will try to match one QRS complex for each P wave. If the atrial rate falls below 60 or it goes above 100, the pacemaker will provide a pre-determined rate of ventricular impulses to maintain circulation. This mechanism is particularly useful in patients with uncontrolled atrial rates where they need to increase their heart rate during physical activity and exertion.

Identifying Paced EKG Rhythm

Pacemaker provides characteristic electronic artifact called **pacer spikes** and is seen in an EKG depending on the chamber paced. For example, if the pacemaker is giving *impulse to atria*, EKG will have pacer spike, which is a straight vertical line *right before the origin of P wave.* Similarly, in *ventricular pacing rhythm, location of pacer spike is right before the QRS*

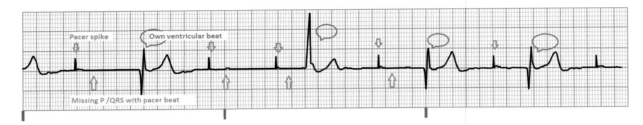

Fig 10.5 Failure to capture

complex. In dual chamber pacemaker, there are *two spikes* positioned one in front of P wave and one for QRS.

It is important to remember that in routine telemetry monitoring, the spikes may not appear if the electronic filter setting to eliminate artifacts is enabled within the computer software. Again, in the new generation bipolar pacemakers, this electrical artifact is less obvious because of the close proximity of both positive and negative poles compared to old generation pacemakers where the lead was considered positive pole and the generator unit was negative.

Complications During Pacemaker Therapy

"Hey, watch out that rhythm in 24. His pacemaker is skipping", Reena said to Joy. *"You have the patient, right?"* Reena continued. *"No, I was covering for Abel when she was on break. He was okay at that time",* Joyce said by pushing her chair towards the telemetry monitoring screen. *"Yeah, I see what you mean. The guy has a temporary. He has sepsis. Lactate was 5 this morning I heard",* Joyce

said by nodding her and continued. "I'll call Abel. She better let Dr. Patel know before we have a disaster", Joy continued while looking for Abel's number on the resource sheet. Joy talked to Abel and discussed about the telemetry findings. She later called the intensivist Dr. Patel on duty and managed the patient.*

Capture Failure

In ideal setting, each pacemaker impulse should produce corresponding P or QRS complex depending on the chamber being paced. In some instances, the EKG will show *pacer spikes at regular intervals* denoting normal functioning pacemaker with *no trailing P or QRS complexes.* Here, the myocardium did not capture the impulse given by the pacemaker.

Common causes for capture failure are (1) *lead malfunction* such as broken or dislodged leads either at myocardium or pacemaker generator level, (2) increased energy requirement for myocardial stimulation (*increased pacer threshold*) secondary to *metabolic or electrolyte imbalance, fibrosis of myocardium* at the site of lead insertion and use of *antiarrhythmic drugs* (increase pacer threshold).

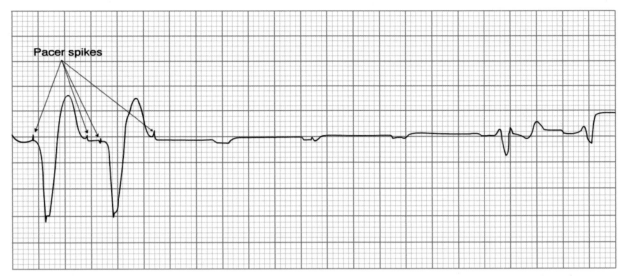

Fig 10.6 Failure to pace

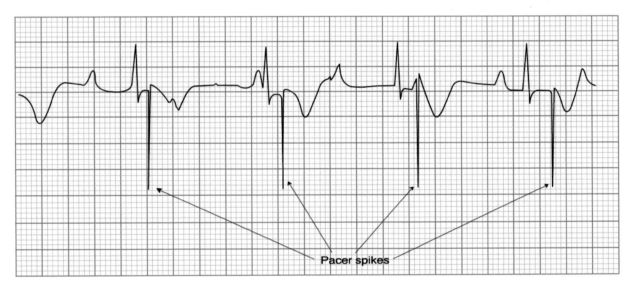

Fig 10.7 Failure to sense

Failure to Pace

This situation is evident in the EKG as *missed beats when pacemaker was supposed to initiate an impulse*. If left untreated, this rhythm is dangerous as it essentially jeopardizes the reason for having a pacemaker at the first place. Probable causes for failure to pace include *weak battery*, *lead failure*, programming issues such as *poor sensing* and *electromagnetic interference (EMI)*.

Failure to Sense (Under Sensing)

Here, the pacemaker *does not sense the intrinsic impulse for which it was supposed to inhibit pacing function*. In EKG, there are *multiple pacer spikes irrespective of the patient's own impulses*. Interestingly, all of these pacer impulses do not generate corresponding cardiac activity because of the **absolute refractory period** within the cardiac cycle. However, if any of these pacer beats happen to strike on the downward slope of T wave, where ventricles are most vulnerable for lethal arrhythmias, ventricular tachycardia may result. This is mostly caused by *under sensing, lead malfunction, electromagnetic interference* etc.

Over Sensing

In this situation, the pacemaker can *misinterpret* muscle movements and normal cardiac waveforms like T wave as innate electrical impulses and can act inappropriately. Misinterpreting T waves as QRS complex and interpreting entire rhythm as tachycardia when the heart rate is within normal limits is commonly seen in high-energy devices like ICD. This is dangerous because these devices are programmed to terminate ventricular tachycardia by override pacing or electrical cardioversion. Therefore, the patient can get inappropriate shock therapy from these devices in these situations. *An appropriate programming change in the devise is* the treatment of choice.

Complications of Pacemaker Implantation

- Infection
- Hematoma
- Pneumothorax
- Cardiac perforation
- Diaphragmatic or phrenic nerve stimulation
- Lead dislodgement
- Skin erosion at implantation site

Box 10.2 Complications of pacemaker implantation

Pacemaker Safety-Patient Education

There are many misconceptions regarding activities and appliances a patient with pacemaker can engage in daily life. It is very important to adequately reassure and inform the patient regarding *do's and don'ts* after having a pacemaker. The most important and serious concern is the possibility of electromagnetic interference (EMI) from adjacent devices.

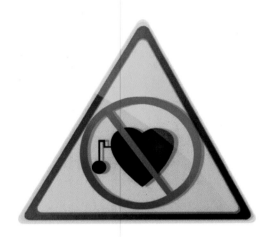

As a matter of fact, the pacemakers have come a long way from their predecessors so that newer generation devices are very much sealed from outside electromagnetic interference generated by day-to-day appliances including cell phones and microwave ovens. Different manufacturers give specifications about their devices however, in general these devices are safe as long as the person who has the pacemaker stays at a reasonable distance from EMI generating devices. Most common *unsafe devises for pacemakers are high-energy electromagnetic devices such as MRI scan, electrical generators, welding equipment* etc.

Points to Remember!!!

- Fixed rate pacemakers provide impulses at a fixed rate irrespective of person's own cardiac activity; however, demand pacemakers generate impulses within a programmed range based on innate cardiac function.

- Depending on the number of chambers sensed or paced, pacemakers can be single or dual chamber.

- In complete heart block dual chamber pacemaker is of great use, since there is no connection between the atria and the ventricle.

- Biventricular pacemakers are used to re-establish synchronization of ventricular contraction.

- Depending on the duration of use, pacemakers can be temporary or permanent.

- Most common complications of temporary pacemaker are infection and lead dislodgement.

- There are different modes of pacing exists based on the chamber's being paced or sensed and the mode of response of pacemaker based on the intrinsic cardiac activity.

- Rate responsiveness allows the pacemakers to respond appropriately in the event of erratic impulse production such as atrial fibrillation.

- Paced EKG rhythm shows the pacemaker spike before P or QRS or both waveforms depending on the chamber being paced.

- Pacer spikes are not visualized in the EKG if the electronic filter setting to eliminate artifacts is enabled.

- Compared to older generation unipolar pacemakers, the spikes produced in newer bipolar pacemakers are relatively small and sometimes not seen in the EKG.

- In 'failure to capture', there will be pacer spikes in EKG with no corresponding QRS complexes.

- Lead malfunction, increased pacer threshold, myocardial fibrosis, use of antiarrhythmic drugs etc. are common causes of capture failure.

- 'Failure to pace' exists when the pacemaker failed to initiate an impulse when it is supposed to do so.

- Lead failure, weak battery, poor sensing and electromagnetic interference are the possible causes of pacing failure.

- When the pacemaker does not recognize innate cardiac activity and provide paced impulses inappropriately, it is called failure to sense or under sensing.

- Pacing in the down slope of T wave can produce polymorphic ventricular tachycardia.

- During over sensing, pacemaker misinterprets tall T waves as QRS complexes and respond as if there is tachycardia exist (essentially double counting QRS complexes and so as the ventricular rate).

- Pacemakers are not safe with high-energy electromagnetic devices such as MRI scan, electrical generators, welding equipment etc. They are pretty safe with the day-to-day household appliance.

Test Your Understanding

1. Which of the following is true regarding fixed rate pacemakers?
A   They provide impulse depending on person's heart rate
B   They provide impulse irrespective of person's heart rate
C   They provide impulse to both atria and ventricle
D   They only have left ventricular lead

2. Which of the following option of pacemaker is ideal for sick sinus syndrome?
A   Fixed the rate of pacemaker
B   Demand pacemakers
C   Biventricular pacemaker
D   Implantable defibrillator

3. Cardiac resynchronization therapy (CRT) is achieved by_____
A   Atrial pacemaker
B   Single chamber ventricular pacemaker
C   Dual chamber demand pacemaker
D   Biventricular pacemaker

4. Which of the following is the most important goal achieved by cardiac resynchronization therapy (CRT)?
A   Re-establishing atrio ventricular synchrony
B   Preserving simultaneous ventricular depolarization
C   Preventing atrio ventricular synchrony
D   Suppressing SA node

5. Which of the following is not a complication of temporary pacemaker implantation?
A   Infection
B   Long-term skin erosion
C   Lead dislodgement
D   Bleeding

6. A permanent pacemaker is not indicated in _____
A   Complete heart block
B   Idioventricular rhythm
C   Symptomatic bradycardia
D   Sinus tachycardia

7. The third letter in pacemaker mode represent_____
A   Chamber paced
B   Chamber sensed
C   Rate response
D   Response to intrinsic rhythm

8. In a DDIR pacemaker mode, second letter D stands for_____
A   Single chamber pacing
B   Single chamber sensing
C   Dual chamber sensing
D   Dual chamber pacing

9. Which of the following situation benefit from rate responsiveness of a pacemaker?
A   Normal sinus rhythm
B   Sinus bradycardia
C   Atrial fibrillation with rapid ventricular response
D   Atrial fibrillation with a controlled ventricular response

10. Which of the following represent 'failure to pace'?
A   Presence of extra beats
B   Missing beats when pacemaker was supposed to fire
C   Presence of pacemaker spike without corresponding rhythm

D   Presence of spike within an intrinsic QRS complex

Answers

1.   B   They provide impulse irrespective of person's heart rate
2.   B   Demand pacemakers
3.   D   Biventricular pacemaker
4.   B   Preserving simultaneous ventricular depolarization
5.   B   Long-term skin erosion
6.   D   Sinus tachycardia
7.   D   Response to intrinsic rhythm
8.   C   Dual chamber sensing
9.   C   Atrial fibrillation with rapid ventricular response
10. C   Presence of pacemaker spike without corresponding rhythm

PART 3

COMPREHENSIVE 12 LEAD EKG ANALYSIS

CHAPTER 11

12 Lead EKG

In this chapter

- Steps in 12 Lead EKG interpretation
- Electrical axis of the heart
- Axis deviation
- Right bundle branch block
- Left anterior and posterior hemiblock
- Left bundle branch block

Clinical scenario

"What is going on? I see you're looking at this EKG for last 10 minutes. Anything interesting?", Leticia asked Mandy. "I'm trying to see whether I can learn to read this EKG. I bought this pocket card the other day. I was using it to identify the rhythm and its characteristics", Mandy replied. "I'm glad you're trying to learn EKG. It is one of the fundamental skills that any nurse working in cardiac or ICU should know of. It can be great use when your patients are in trouble. This looks like a good tool" Leticia said. "I'm trying to learn the methods so that I can confidently read EKG's", Mandy said. "Doesn't matter what tool you use. You have to do it in a systematic way so that you don't miss any vital information", Leticia, one of the veteran ICU nurses replied by flipping through the pages of EKG pocket tool that Mandy handed over to her.

Then she continued "I don't recommend you looking at the machine interpretation that comes with the 12 lead EKG. I prefer you learn the technique by analyzing yourself the characteristics of the rhythm. Also make sure you evaluate all the limb leads, augmented leads and precordial leads in the rhythm. Remember, you're looking at the electrical activity of a three-dimensional structure through the EKG. So, you have to look through multiple angles to get the real story".

A 12-lead electrocardiogram is essentially the most affordable, accessible and basic diagnostic evaluation that provides a comprehensive view of the electrical activity in the heart. As we discussed in earlier chapters, individual leads provide only a single view of the three-dimensional heart. Since we are trying to recreate a two-dimensional image of the three-dimensional structure as the heart, we must put together all the available views that provide maximum amount of information. In a 12 lead EKG, the leads are generally grouped together based on the representation of different walls of the heart. Combination of limb leads (lead I, II and III), augmented leads (aVR, aVL, aVF) and precordial leads (V1-V6) are generally used in identification of underlying physiologic processes.

P wave, **QRS** complex, **T** wave and *their characteristics* and *morphology. Heart rate, various intervals* and *presence of any ectopic beats* should be noted. Some 12 lead EKG machines provide two or more running leads along with regular 12 leads, which help in identifying basic characteristics.

2. **Determine overall axis**: Electrical axis of the EKG simply shows the *direction of electricity flow* within the heart. Normally it is directed towards left and inferior aspect of the heart (towards left ventricle). Any defects in normal conduction pattern such as bundle branch block and chamber thickness (hypertrophy) changes overall axis of the EKG.

3. **Presence of block**: Assess for **bundle branch block** or **hemiblock.**

4. Check for **chamber enlargement** or thickness (Hypertrophy).

Steps in 12 Lead EKG Interpretation

A systematic approach should be used similar to a single lead interpretation while accessing a 12 lead EKG. This method will prevent overlooking any information that could be vital in diagnosis and treatment of a given patient. Important steps are as follows

1. **Determine the rhythm**: Just like assessing a single lead EKG, *look for the presence of*

Steps in 12 lead EKG Interpretation

1. **R**hythm

2. **A**xis

3. **B**undle branch block

4. **E**nlargement of chamber

5. **I**schemia or infarction

6. **O**ther abnormalities

Box 11.1 **Steps in EKG interpretation**

5. Check for **ischemia** or **infarction**

6. Look for **other abnormalities** like hyperkalemia, A-V dissociation etc.

Clinical scenario

"Would you please explain to me what meant by axis of the heart? I tried to read it. But it doesn't make much sense to me" Mandy, who is a student nurse asked Leticia. "Well, remember that I told you before, the heart is a three-dimensional organ and has electricity moving through the tissue that causes contraction. So, when electricity goes through a three-dimensional structure it can go in three different dimensions X, Y and Z axis. Electrical axis simply means the direction of electricity flow within the heart. In general, more electricity goes towards the biggest muscle mass within the heart. That happens to be towards the left ventricle. If you look at the EKG, you can see the net direction of this electricity and is called normal axis", Leticia replied by pointing to the picture in the EKG pocket tool. "So, what could change the direction of electricity within the heart?" Mandy asked. "There are many reasons", Leticia continued, "There are different kinds of axis deviation like right axis deviation, left axis deviation and indeterminant axis deviation. Any abnormal electric circuits, change in muscle mass of the heart like hypertrophy, myocardial infarction and so forth can cause change in electrical axis".

Electrical Axis of the Heart

Electrical axis simply means, *overall direction of the electrical flow within the heart.* As we discussed earlier, in a normal heart the electrical impulse starts from the **SA node**, travels down to the **AV node** and then spreads across the ventricles through **Purkinje fibers**. As the *left ventricle is the major pumping chamber and having the greatest muscle thickness, much of this current flows towards left ventricle* with an effective **leftward and downward** direction. This direction is also known as **leftward and inferior** and is **the normal axis** of the EKG. Any defects in electrical circuit changes the direction of electric flow and thereby the axis. Therefore, axis determination helps in identifying *structural and electrophysiologic defects* in the heart.

Some of the basic concepts of EKG are very valuable in identifying the axis and understanding other major concepts in 12 lead interpretation process.

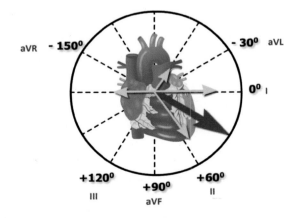

Fig 11.1 Mean electrical axis of the heart

Two most important basic concepts are

1. Electricity flowing *towards positive electrode* generate a *positive (upright)* deflection in the resulting EKG
2. Individual lead in an EKG provides **single linear view** of electrical activity of the heart.

Application of these basic principles to the conceptual diagram developed by the Nobel Prize winner William Einthoven helps to identify clinical significance of various leads in a 12 lead EKG.

Visualizing Axis in the Frontal Plane

Lead **I**, **II**, **III**, **aVR**, **aVL** and **aVF** constitute the **frontal plane leads** in a 12 lead EKG. Precordial leads **V1** to **V6** provide *horizontal plane view of the heart*. Among the frontal leads, lead

Causes of Axis Deviation

Right Axis Deviation
Normal variation in children and thin adults
Chronic lung disease
WPW syndrome
Left posterior hemiblock
Antero lateral MI
Right ventricular hypertrophy

Left Axis Deviation
Normal variation in obesity, pregnancy and ascites
Left anterior hemiblock
Inferior wall MI
Left ventricular hypertrophy
Premature ventricular contraction

Indeterminant Axis Deviation
Premature ventricular contraction

Box 11.2 Causes of axis deviation

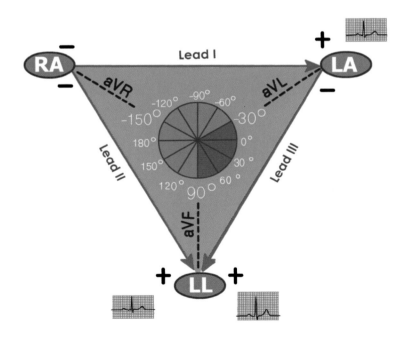

Fig 11.2 Frontal leads with their positive electrodes

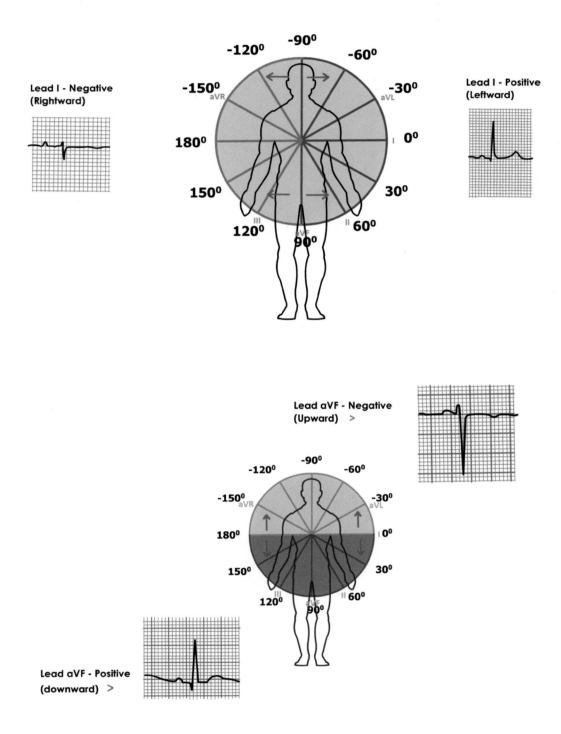

Fig 11.3 Lead I and aVF with their waveform and corresponding direction

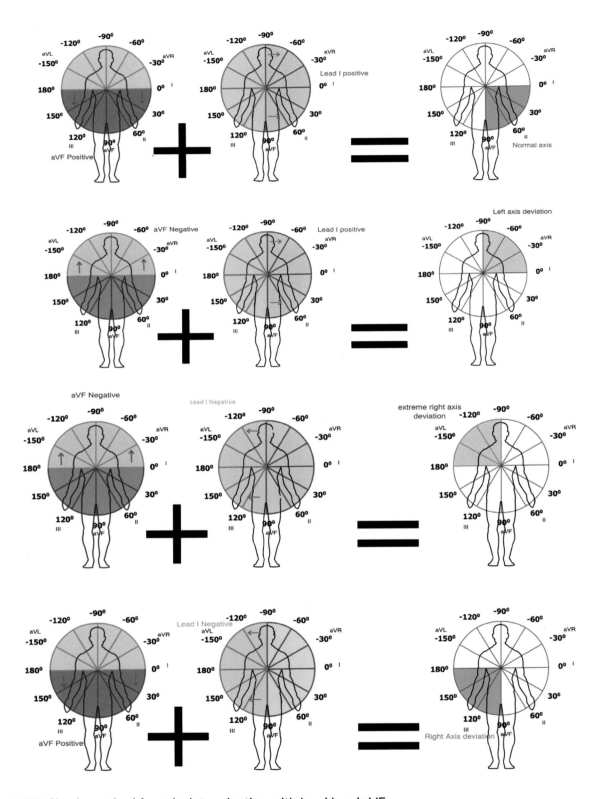

Fig 11.3 B Simple method for axis determination with Lead I and aVF

Simple Method for Right or Left Axis Determination

Lead	Normal Axis	Right axis deviation	Left axis deviation
I	Positive	Negative	Positive
II	Positive	Positive or Negative	Negative
III	Positive or Negative	Positive	Negative
aVF	Positive	Positive	Negative

Box 11.3 Right and left axis determination

I has a positive electrode on the left shoulder and negative electrode on the right. In lead **I** an electrical activity travelling *towards left* will generate a *positive deflection* in the resulting EKG. Hence, lead **I** can be used in *differentiating impulses going towards* **left** (EKG with a positive wave) *from that going towards* **right** (a negative wave).

Similarly, lead **aVF** has a positive electrode on the left lower extremity. Lead aVF can be used to differentiate electricity going towards *up* or *downward direction*. Even though a bit confusing, it is important to recall the principle that when electricity flows downward (towards positive electrode), it produces a positive waveform in lead **aVF**. Remember, lead aVF has positive electrode on the left lower end of the body and the direction of current is towards this positive electrode. Conversely when **aVF** is negative, it denotes electricity flowing in upward direction.

The rest of the limbs leads are shown in this diagram (Fig 11.2). The diagram also shows direction of QRS complex depending on whether the impulses travel towards or away from them. Even though lead **I** and **aVF** are the initial leads we assess in order to get a general orientation of the axis, other augmented and limb leads help to pinpoint the axis within this diagram.

Major emphasize has given to the topic of axis determination and direction of electrical forces in this session as they serve as the foundation for the rest of EKG analysis including identification of bundle branch block.

Once the vertical axis is determined, it is important to see the direction of electricity in the horizontal plane. In a normal heart the direction of flow of current is towards the left ventricle and that is towards posterior (Remember, anatomically right ventricle is more towards the anterior chest wall. Compared to the right ventricle, the left ventricle is situated more posteriorly). Flow of current in posterior direction is shown by a positive wave in lead **V6**, which is closer to the left ventricle (Remember the position of **V6** electrode).

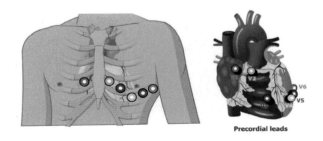

Precordial leads

Fig 11.4 Precordial leads in relation to heart

Since lead **V1** and **V2** are situated in the anterior aspect of the chest wall, any flow of current in the anterior direction results in a positive waveform in these leads. The precordial leads are arranged in an *anterior to posterior* fashion so that they help to pinpoint the direction of electrical flow in the horizontal plane.

Coronary Circulation to the Conduction System

Conduction system tissues receive blood through various branches of right and left coronary arteries. In general, right coronary artery (RCA) supplies blood to the proximal part of the conduction system including SA node and AV node. Left anterior descending artery (LAD) provides supply to middle and distal aspects of the conduction system. As a failsafe mechanism, some of the key elements of conduction system receive *dual blood supply* from two different arteries to ensures adequate function of these areas in the event of the compromise of any one of the arteries.

The Sino atrial node (SA node) is predominantly supplied by branch of right coronary artery called **SA nodal branch**. The *AV node and bundle of his receive dual blood supply from both the right coronary artery (RCA) and branch of left anterior descending artery (LAD). Left circumflex artery provides blood supply to the posterior fascicle of left bundle branch.* The distal aspect of the bundle branch like *right bundle branch and anterior fascicle of left bundle branch receive blood supply from the left anterior descending artery.*

Adequate understanding of the relation between coronary blood supply and conduction system is very important. Occlusion of any of these arteries or branches can cause corresponding electrical abnormality in the EKG. It also explains the importance of looking for specific types of arrhythmias including bundle branch block, fascicular block or complete heart block in the event of occlusion of different coronary arteries.

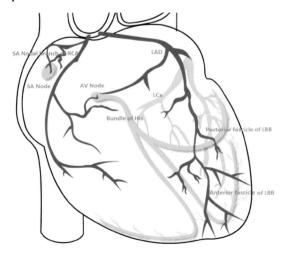

Fig 11.4 B Coronary blood supply to the conduction system

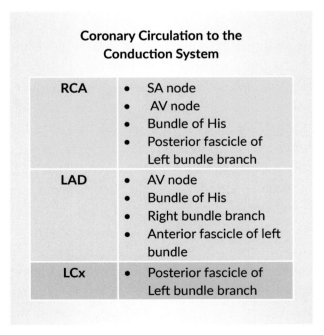

Coronary Circulation to the Conduction System	
RCA	• SA node • AV node • Bundle of His • Posterior fascicle of Left bundle branch
LAD	• AV node • Bundle of His • Right bundle branch • Anterior fascicle of left bundle
LCx	• Posterior fascicle of Left bundle branch

Box 11.4 Coronary circulation to the conduction system

"Pardon me if I'm asking a stupid question", Mandy said to John. "There is no question called stupid question. When you're asking a question that means you're not stupid". John turned around with a smile while trying to disconnect an IV line from the bedside pump. "Okay, is this ventricular tachycardia?" Mandy asked pointing to the bedside monitor. "No, absolutely not". John continued, "I know why you had that question. You're looking at a wide complex rhythm, correct?" John asked. "Yes, yes. When I looked at it I thought the wide QRS indicate ventricular tachycardia", Mandy replied. "Mr. Rodriguez has a bundle branch block. That is why the QRS is wider than usual, give me a second", John then turned around and asked the patient. "Mr. Rodriguez, is there anything else I can do for you when I'm here now?". "No, I'm okay. Do you know when the doctor is coming?", The patient asked. "Sorry, I don't know exactly. Is there anything that you want to ask the doctor? I can page him if you want", John replied. "No, nothing important. I just want to know when I can go home", patient said. "You know you came with bad pneumonia, correct?", John asked. "Yes, I know", patient continued. "I hope I get to go home soon". "Yeah, maybe in few days. You need some heavy-duty antibiotic before going home so that you don't have to come back again, right?" John continued, "Ok, I'll be back in half an hour. If there is anything press the call button", John said while walking out of the room. "Let's go and look at his EKG rhythm strip", John said to Mandy.

Right Bundle Branch Block

In normal electrical conduction system, impulses traveling down from the AV node take the path of least resistance, which is the bundle of his. These impulses then travel to the left and right bundle branches to spread throughout the ventricle. *Right ventricle is supplied by the right bundle branch* and *left ventricle by anterior and posterior fascicle of the left bundle* branch.

When the right bundle is blocked, the only way right ventricle can get an impulse is from the left ventricle. However, the delay in conduction of impulse from left ventricle to the right ventricle causes the ventricles to contract *sequentially* (back to back) *rather than simultaneously* (together).

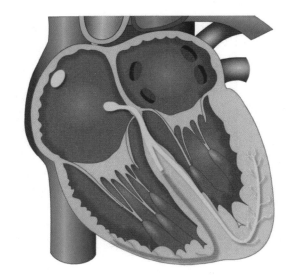

Fig 11.5 Conduction system with RBBB

This process may affect the hemodynamics because of the impaired movement of Inter ventricular septum. In this situation, *the last part of QRS complex* will be directing towards *right ventricle, which is* **anterior** *and right-ward* instead of *left ventricle that is leftward and posterior.*

Lead **I**, **V1** and **V6** are considered in identifying **right bundle branch block (RBBB)**. *The hallmark of any bundle branch block is a wide QRS complex with duration greater than 0.12 seconds.* If the duration is between 0.10 seconds to the 0.11, it is called **Inter ventricular conduction delay** (**IVCD**).

> Observation of the **last half of QRS** complex helps to identify bundle branch block in an EKG. This is different from the evaluation of entire QRS complex to evaluate axis determination.

In right bundle branch block, the net direction of flow of current is towards right ventricle, which is *anterior and rightward.* Therefore, along with a wide QRS complex of duration greater than 0.12 seconds, *lead I and V6 will be*

negative and *lead V1 will be positive* as shown in Fig 11.6. Because of the characteristic electricity flow of bundle branch block in general, **T waves are in opposite direction of QRS complex.** In an EKG with the right bundle branch block, *it is important to evaluate* **overall axis, ST segment elevation, myocardial infarction** and presence of **hemiblock.** Since the contraction of right bundle is sequential, this EKG is *not reliable for identifying right ventricle hypertrophy.*

> Criteria for right bundle branch block include wide QRS complex with duration **greater than 0.12** seconds, **negative** lead I, V6 and **positive** lead **V1.**

Left Hemiblock (Left Anterior Superior Hemiblock)

Left bundle has two distinct bundle segments called left **anterior** or **superior fascicle** and left **posterior fascicle.** During *left anterior hemiblock, left anterior fascicle is blocked.* In order

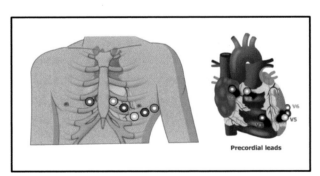

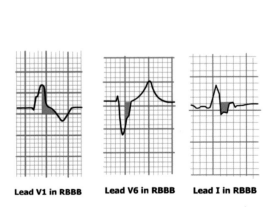

Lead V1 in RBBB   **Lead V6 in RBBB**   **Lead I in RBBB**

Fig 11.6 B Frontal and precordial plane EKG in RBBB (Note the shaded areas under consideration for evaluation of bundle branch block)

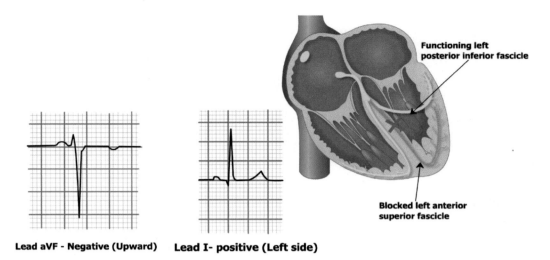

Lead aVF - Negative (Upward)   Lead I- positive (Left side)

Fig 11.7 left anterior hemiblock direction

to depolarize areas of myocardium covered by the anterior fascicle, the impulses spreading through posterior fascicle travel upward (towards anterior).

This upward movement of current changes the axis of EKG in the frontal plane as evidenced by a negative aVF (remember, negative aVF means upward direction of current as aVF has positive electrode towards left leg). The mean direction of QRS in LAHB is therefore leftward and upward.

Since part of the left bundle is still functioning, there *will not be any widening of QRS complex.* However, this EKG may have a slight slurring of the QRS complex called delayed intrinsicoid deflection where the time taken for the R wave to peak from the beginning of the QRS will be longer than usual (>0.45 Sec or greater than 1 small box). Left anterior hemiblock is also known as left anterior superior hemiblock. Left anterior hemiblock has left axis deviation since aVL is positive and lead II, III and aVF are negative.

In left inferior or posterior hemiblock, the direction of current will be from the anterior fascicle to the posterior fascicle and therefore

EKG criteria for left anterior hemiblock are

- **Positive** lead I (leftward) and **negative aVF** (upward) (Left axis deviation)
- qR complex in lateral limb leads (Lead I and aVL)
- qS complex in inferior leads (Lead II, III and aVF)
- Delayed intrinsicoid deflection

rightward and inferior. So, lead I and aVL are negative (rightward), lead II, III and aVF are positive (Inferior or downward). Lead aVR is mostly isoelectric, showing its perpendicular direction with the axis of EKG.

EKG criteria for left posterior hemiblock are

- **Negative** Lead I and positive **aVF** (Right axis deviation)
- rS pattern in lateral limb leads (Lead I and aVL)
- Tall R waves in inferior leads (Lead II, III and aVF- goes with right axis)
- Looks like **S1Q3T3** pattern of EKG findings in **pulmonary embolism**

Left Bundle Branch Block

As mentioned earlier, the right ventricle is supplied by the right bundle branch and the left ventricle by anterior and posterior fascicles of the left bundle branch. In **left bundle branch block**, *the main left bundle before it's bifurcation in to anterior and posterior fascicle is blocked*.

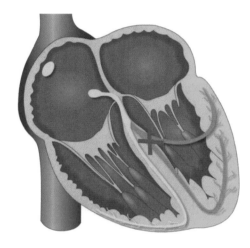

Fig 11.8-Left bundle branch block (Involving both fascicles of Left bundle branch)

This prevents a large area of myocardium in the left ventricle to receive electrical impulse through the conventional route. Here, right ventricle contracts first because of the electric impulse through intact right bundle.

Then the same impulse travels to the left ventricular myocardium, causing it to contract. Therefore, during left bundle branch block the right and left ventricles contract *sequentially rather than in tandem*.

Because of the depolarization of right bundle branch before that of the left bundle, areas of the heart including Inter-ventricular septum that are supplied by the right bundle, contracts inward into the right ventricle during right bundle depolarization. Subsequently it remains dyskinetic during the sequential left ventricular depolarization. This paradoxical movement reduces capacity of left ventricle to pump blood out in to the aorta during systole and cause hemodynamic instability in certain patients. In this situation, the direction of current is from

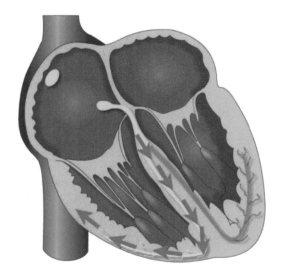

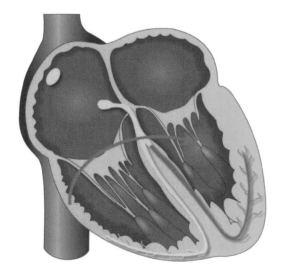

Fig 11.9 LBBB ventricular contraction

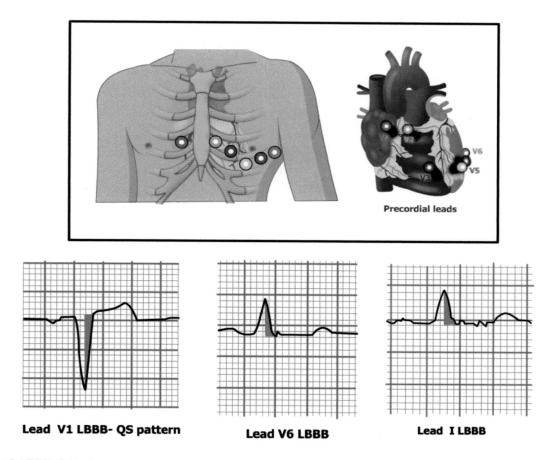

Lead V1 LBBB- QS pattern

Lead V6 LBBB

Lead I LBBB

Fig 11.10 LBBB Criteria

the right ventricle to the left and therefore the last half of QRS direction is towards patient's **left side and posterior**. (Remember, during assessment of bundle branch block we only look at the second half of QRS complex and its direction).

Similar to the right bundle branch block, the direction of T wave is opposite to that of QRS complex in left bundle block. Because of the abnormal formation of QRS, LBBB EKG is not reliable to measure ischemia, infarction, hemiblock or hypertrophy.

For summery of 12 lead interpretation, please refer to the Appendix A

EKG criteria for **LBBB** are **positive ending** of lead **I** and **V6** (R or R'), **QS wave** in lead **V1** and wide QRS complex with duration greater than 0.12 seconds

Points to Remember!!!

- A 12 lead EKG provides three-dimensional view of electrical activity of the heart.
- For accurate interpretation of 12 lead EKG, a stepwise process with

identification of rhythm, axis, presence of bundle branch block, chamber enlargement, presence of ischemic changes and other abnormalities needs to be followed.

- Electrical axis represents overall direction of electrical flow within the heart. Normally, it is directed towards left and inferior, i.e. towards left ventricle.

- Presence of structural or electrophysiologic abnormalities may change normal electrical axis.

- Electricity flows towards positive electrode generate positive deflection in the resulting EKG.

- Chronic lung disease, right ventricular hypertrophy, WPW syndrome, anterolateral myocardial infarction etc. are the common reasons for right axis deviation.

- Left axis deviation is seen in left anterior hemiblock, PVC, inferior wall MI etc.

- Left axis deviation is a normal variant in obese or pregnant individuals.

- Premature ventricular contraction may produce in determinant axis.

- A positive waveform in lead I shows the leftward direction of current.

- Positive waveform in lead aVF represents downward direction of current.

- Lead I and aVF are used primarily for gross determination of axis.

- In normal axis, lead I and aVF will be positive.

- In right bundle branch block, the contractions of ventricles are sequential rather than simultaneous.

- The direction of current in right bundle branch block is anterior and rightward.

- For assessing bundle branch block, only the last half of QRS complex needs to be analyzed.

- In right bundle branch block (RBBB), Lead V1 has a positive ending QRS and lead V6 and I have negative waves as the last half of QRS.

- Wide QRS complex with duration from 0.10 to 0.11 is called inter ventricular conduction delay (IVCD).

- In right bundle branch block EKG; the rhythm can be further analyzed for ischemia, infarction or presence of hemiblock.

- Right bundle branch block pattern is not reliable for assessing right ventricular hypertrophy.

- In hemiblock pattern, there is no widening of QRS complex.

- Left anterior hemiblock changes overall axis of QRS to left and upward direction, creating positive lead I and negative aVF.

- In left posterior or inferior hemiblock, the direction of current is inferior and rightward resulting in negative lead I and aVL with positive lead II, III and aVF.

- In left bundle branch block, overall direction of current is towards left and posterior, resulting in an EKG with positive ending lead I and V6 and negative V1.

- In bundle branch block pattern, the direction of T wave is opposite to that of QRS complex because of the disorganized repolarization.

- Left bundle branch block pattern EKG is not reliable for assessing ischemic changes.

Test Your Understanding

1. Which of the following is an example for the augmented lead?
A   Lead III
B   Lead V6
C   Lead aVR
D   Lead V3

2. 12 lead EKG interpretation can provide information except_____?
A   Thickness of ventricular wall
B   Presence of ischemia
C   Rate of flow through mitral valve
D   Atrioventricular synchronization

3. Based on the principle of direction of current and morphology of waveform, which of the following represent direction of current towards left side of the heart?
A   Positive lead aVL
B   Negative lead V1
C   Positive lead I
D   Negative lead I

4. Which of the following lead is useful in identifying direction of electricity upward or downward?
A   Lead aVR
B   Lead aVL
C   Lead I
D   Lead aVF

5. Which of the following precordial lead has a characteristic tall R wave when electricity is flowing towards left and posterior direction?
A   Lead V1
B   Lead V3
C   Lead V2
D   Lead V6

6. Which of the following is not a characteristic of right bundle branch block?
A   QRS duration 0.18 second
B   QRS duration 0.14 seconds
C   Positive ending lead V6
D   Positive ending of lead V1

7. Which of the following pathology cannot be assessed from right bundle branch block EKG?
A   ST segment elevation
B   Left posterior hemiblock
C   Left ventricular hypertrophy
D   Right ventricular hypertrophy

8. Which of the following statement is true regarding left bundle branch block?
A   Even though hemiblock cannot be assessed, ischemic changes are evident in LBBB
B   Presence of R or R' in lead I and V6 are characteristic of LBBB
C   QRS duration is always greater than 0.18 second in LBBB
D   Direction of current flow in LBBB is towards rightward and anterior

9. What is the main difference in method of identifying the axis deviation and bundle branch block from an EKG?
A   For axis deviation, consider only first-half of QRS complex whereas in BBB, the entire complex
B   In axis deviation, the entire wave to be considered whereas in BBB, only lasts half of QRS
C   In BBB, first-half of QRS is under consideration whereas in axis deviation, entire PQRST complex to be considered
D   In BBB, QRS complex in the beginning and end of the rhythm is considered

10. Which of the following is not a characteristic of left anterior superior hemiblock?

A   Direction of current towards leftward and upward

B   QRS duration greater than 0.12 second

C   It has positive lead I

D   There is negative aVF

Answers

1.   C   Lead aVR

2.   C   Rate of flow through mitral valve

3.   C   Positive lead I

4.   D   Lead aVF

5.   D   Lead V6

6.   C   Positive ending lead V6

7.   D   Right ventricular hypertrophy

8.   B   Presence of R or R' in lead I and V6 are characteristic of LBBB

9.   B   In axis deviation, the entire wave to be considered whereas in BBB, only lasts half of QRS

10. B.   QRS duration greater than 0.12 seconds

CHAPTER 12

Myocardial Ischemia and Infarction

In this chapter

- Pathophysiology of Myocardial infarction
- 12 lead EKG and coronary distribution
- Diagnostic value of 12 lead EKG
- Types of myocardial events
- EKG criteria for various events

Clinical scenario

"How can we help you, sir?". Arlene asked while walking into the patient's room with Michelle who is a student nurse. "I'm feeling some heaviness in my chest the last 10 minutes. I thought it was gas. Now it feels like getting worse", patient replied. "Huh, let's see", Arlene said and continued. "How bad is the pain now?". "It's not pain, I feel some heavy ..." Patient paused and then continued, "I feel like something sitting on my chest". "Okay, that doesn't sound right. You also look little sweaty, let's get the EKG machine over here. Michelle, can you please go and get the EKG machine right by the crash cart? You know where it is, right?" Arlene asked Michelle. "I know, I'll be right back", Michelle said and walked out of the room. When Michelle came back with the machine, Arlene already had 2 other ICU nurses at bedside. One of them hooked the EKG leads. The patient is already on oxygen. "Here is the morphine that you asked", charge nurse Joel said by walking in to the room with a medicine

cartridge in hand. "Okay folks, activate STEMI. looks like inferior", Melinda, who was another ICU nurse in the room said with an alarming voice after looking at 12 lead EKG rhythm. The patient was immediately taken to the Cath Lab for coronary intervention. After the patient had gone for the procedure, Michelle asked Arlene. "So, I heard Melinda saying it is STEMI and inferior. What is it exactly mean?". "Well... there are different kinds of myocardial infarction. An acute closure of coronary artery can cause ST elevation myocardial infarction with the characteristic changes in the EKG corresponding to the area affected. For this patient, the changes were in the inferior wall of the heart. That is why she said inferior STEMI. Usually the changes are seen in lead II, III and aVF for inferior STEMI", Arlene replied.

The 12 lead EKG has been a cornerstone diagnostic test for evaluation and treatment of patients with myocardial ischemia and infarction in a timely fashion. Widespread availability, minimal expertise for interpretation and instantaneous result presentation have made the 12 lead EKG one of the most widely used clinical diagnostic tool in modern medicine.

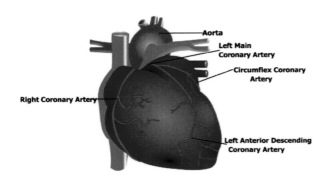

Fig 12.1 Coronary anatomy

Atherosclerotic heart disease (ASHD) accounts for majority of myocardial ischemia and infarction in adult population. Commonly, advanced atherosclerotic heart disease produces a constellation of symptoms known as

Acute Coronary Syndrome (**ACS**) and ST elevation myocardial infarction (**STEMI**).

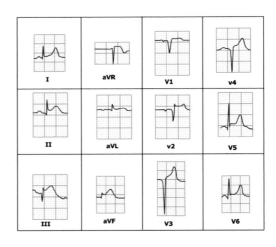

Fig 12.2 ST segment elevation in various leads

However, the most common myocardial ischemic event that come across in real world is Stable Angina Pectoris, characterized by *chest pain* typically *initiated by exertion* either physical or emotional that is *relieved with either rest or use of nitroglycerin*. The characteristics of pain include *squeezing, central* or *sub sternal discomfort* (*Levine's sign*) with the *crescendo decrescendo type* (waxing and waning). The pain usually lasts for *2 to 5 min* with *radiation*

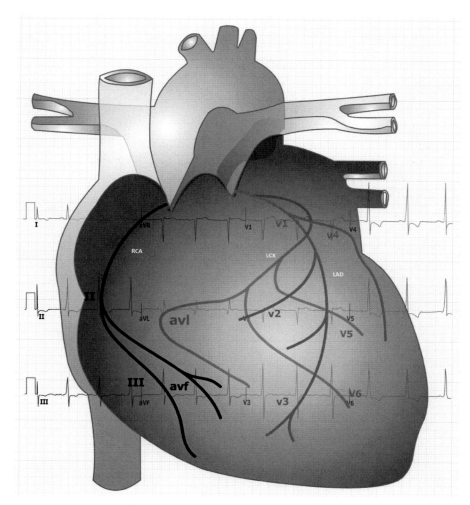

Fig 12.2-B Coronary anatomy and distribution of EKG leads

to *shoulder*, *arm*, *jaw* or *back*. Patient may also have nocturnal angina and demonstrate considerable difference in symptoms through the course of the day because of the variations in coronary vascular tone.

Acute coronary syndrome includes two distinct categories of disease process classified based on the presentation, known as Unstable Angina (UA) and Non-ST Segment Elevation Myocardial Infarction (NSTEMI).

Unstable Angina (**UA**): Here, the patient presents with *unprovoked typical cardiac chest pain* with or without radiation to adjacent areas, may or may not *relieved by rest or sublingual* *nitroglycerin* treatment. These patients may not have any EKG changes or elevation in their target cardiac enzymes such as Troponin I, Creatine phosphokinase (CK) or Creatine phosphokinase-cardiac fraction (CKMB).

Non-ST Segment Elevation Myocardial Infarction (**NSTEMI**): In these patients, along with *anginal symptoms* there may be *ST segment depression or T wave inversion* and *has positive cardiac biomarkers* such as troponin I and CKMB. Sometimes ST segment changes are transient (short lasting).

ST Segment Elevation Myocardial Infarction (**STEMI**): This acute form of myocardial infarction results from *complete and sudden occlusion of a coronary artery* leading to *acute myocardial injury.* This scenario is characterized by consistent *ST segment elevation greater than 0.1 mV* (larger than one small vertical box in an EKG) in two or more contiguous leads in an EKG or *new onset of left bundle branch block* (LBBB) pattern along with angina. There may be coexisting **mirror image changes** in the form of *ST segment depression and T wave inversion* in the areas of EKG opposite to that of ischemia.

In a 12 lead EKG, ST segment changes are consistent with *area of myocardium supplied by the blocked coronary artery.* For example, in anterior wall STEMI the affected vessel is most likely **left anterior descending artery (LAD)** and is evidenced in an EKG by consistent ST segment elevation in lead **V2, V3** and **V4** which are looking at electrical activity on the anterior chest wall. There may also be ST segment depression and T wave inversion in inferior leads **II, III** and **aVF**, which are on the opposite side of the anterior wall. ST segment changes happen because of the *abnormal electrical transmission and subsequent repolarization in chemically unstable environment that exists in ischemic and infarcted myocardium.*

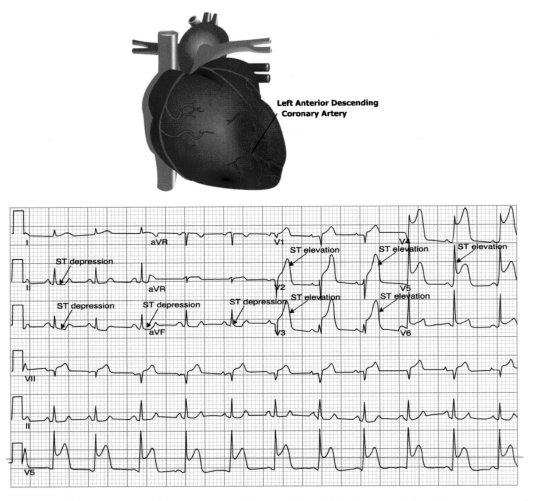

Fig 12.3 Anterior STEMI showing LAD occlusion with resulting EKG changes. (Note the presence of anterior ST elevation and inferior St segment depression changes (Mirror image).

An important principle in diagnosing myocardial events from a 12 lead EKG is that presence of characteristic ST elevation, ST depression, T wave inversion or Q wave in *isolated leads are of least diagnostic significance*. In order to be clinically relevant, these changes have to be seen in contiguous (neighboring) EKG leads.

For example, presence of **Q** wave in lead **III** alone does not indicate inferior wall ischemia without corresponding **Q** wave in lead **II** and **aVF**. This is of extremely important while reporting EKG finding in clinical situations.

Clinical scenario

"Wow, this is crazy". Shane said by looking into the shift report sheet. He then looked at Jane, the night shift ICU nurse and Carla, who is a student nurse. Shane continued, "this guy is only 39 years old, had a massive heart attack?". "Did you ask him what's going on? Is he a heavy guy?". "Sorry I didn't get the time to ask him so much. My bed 23 was all night code brown and confused. So, I was busy with him and his family, both going nuts all night long. Oh boy, I'm exhausted", Jane said with a deep sigh. "Okay, no problem. Me and Carla will figure it out", Shane replied. The day went on. Carla and Shane worked together to take care of their patients in the intensive care unit. By midafternoon, both sat together, and Shane was finishing up documentation on an admission came from the ED. Shane asked Carla "well, did your investigative work turn up anything for our young guy with MI? Did you find what is going on?" "I asked him", Carla continued, "He used to smoke, 1 to 2 cigarettes a day for around 5 years while he was a teenager. He hasn't smoked for last 15 years. He worked as a computer professional. He said his dad had heart attack at the age of 51 and died from it. He is so worried about it". 'Yup... That is something that he needs to be worried of", Shane replied with a deep sigh. "Family history of premature heart disease is a significant risk factor. Yes, smoking, working as a computer professional with sitting all day…", Shane paused and then continued. "What else? I think those are the most important one for him. Do you know anything about his cholesterol?", Shane asked Carla. "He told me, his family has a history of high cholesterol. He was told 3 years ago by his doctor that his cholesterol is high", Carla replied. "Well, that somewhat explains. He has multiple risk factors for coronary artery disease. You know about modifiable and nonmodifiable risk factors for CAD, right?" Shane asked. "I remember hearing about them in the class", Carla said. "There are both modifiable and nonmodifiable risk factors that can contribute to development of atherosclerosis. The stuff that you can work on like… Diabetes, high cholesterol, sedentary lifestyle, smoking and so forth comes in modifiable risk factors. Things like your family history, getting older and similar happen to be in the nonmodifiable risk factor group", Shane continued. "So, for this guy, he has a bad family history and lifestyle. Look at him, he is heavy, right?" Shane asked Carla. "Yes, he is obese", Carla replied. "Risk factor modification is a major aspect of preventing further heart attacks. He has a lot of work to do", Shane said while looking at the computer.

Pathophysiology of ASHD

The core of pathophysiology of atherosclerotic heart disease is a *disparity in supply and demand of myocardial oxygen*. In normal circumstances, epicardial coronary arteries supply enough blood to support oxygen and nutrient demands of myocardial cells depending on the cardiac workload. In ischemic heart disease, because of the narrowing of coronary arteries, some areas of myocardium deprive of adequate blood flow leading to ischemia and infarction.

Major determinants of myocardial oxygen demand (MVO2) are *heart rate, myocardial contractility* and *myocardial wall tension*. In normal disease-free heart, the coronary circulation including micro vascular structures are very effective in adapting to the changing needs of heart to ensure adequate myocardial nutrient supply. However, in coronary artery disease the system lacks flexibility and adaptability for changing needs of the heart. Other factors that can adversely affect coronary blood supply are *arterial thrombi, coronary vessel spasm, emboli* and *severe anemia*.

Coronary atherosclerosis may be produced by factors such as *increased LDL* (Low density lipoprotein), *low HDL* (High density lipoprotein), *smoking, hypertension, diabetes mellitus* etc. These oxidative events disturb normal function of coronary endothelium, leading to local inflammatory changes along with abnormal cell adhesion and plaque buildup. These chronic changes ultimately produce widespread coronary atherosclerosis.

Generally, **50%** reduction in lumen size produces **exercise-induced symptoms** and when reaches greater than **80%**, patient will have **non-exertional symptoms**. Severity of symptoms, extent of myocardial damage and possible treatment options are largely depending on factors like distribution of atherosclerosis in the coronary system, location and extent of disease, presence of alternate pathways or collateral circulation and the timeframe for development of occlusion (acute versus chronic).

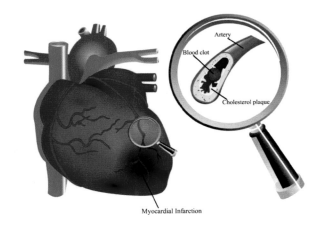

Fig 12.4 Pathophysiology of STEMI

Myocardial oxygen deprivation will produce decreased pH, impaired cell membrane function and similar changes at the cellular level. If the *ischemia continues for more than 20 min, cell death and subsequent scarring of cells (infarction) happens* in the absence of collateral circulation. Ischemia may cause repolarization abnormalities leading to elevation of ST segment, premature beats including ventricular tachycardia and fibrillation.

Evidence has shown that atherosclerotic changes may develop even before the age of 20 and the patients are asymptomatic for a long duration. Ischemic changes also can damage left ventricular myocardium, resulting in heart failure secondary to ischemic cardiomyopathy.

Coronary Circulation and 12 Lead EKG

Leads	Anatomical area	Coronary artery
I, aVL, V5, V6	Lateral wall	Circumflex artery
II, III, aVF	Inferior wall	Right coronary artery
V1, V2	Septum	Left anterior descending artery
V3, V4	Anterior wall	Left anterior descending artery

Box 12.1 EKG leads corresponding to anatomical areas of heart

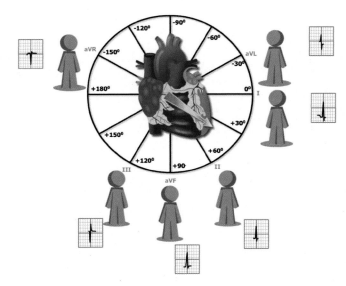

Fig 12.5 12 lead EKG in relation to views of the heart

Common Differential Diagnosis of Chest Pain

- Aortic stenosis
- Cardiomyopathy
- Coronary vasospasm (Printzmetal's angina)
- Cardiac Syndrome X
- Pericarditis
- Aortic dissection
- Cocaine use
- Anemia
- Esophageal diseases
- Pneumonia
- Costochondritis (Tsetse's syndrome)

Box 12.2 Major differentials for chest pain

Diagnostic Testing for Chest Pain

EKG: 12 lead EKG may be normal or with presence of conduction deficits, ST depression and T wave inversions, left ventricular hypertrophy changes etc., unless patient is having a true STEMI.

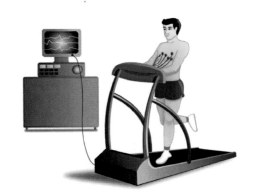

Fig 12.6 Exercise treadmill testing

Exercise stress test: Either physical or chemical stress testing brings out stress induced ischemic changes that are usually *reversible in nature*. Typical *positive ST segment response* is indicated by a *flat or down sloping depression of ST segment* for more than **0.1 mV** below baseline. The study also considered positive in events like hypotensive response to exercise and sustained ventricular arrhythmia induced by stress.

Chemical stress testing with the use of Dipyridamole, Adenosine and Regadenosine (**Lexiscan**) that are vasodilators, combined with nuclear imaging is particularly useful in patients with the left bundle branch block and pacemaker rhythms where EKG is not a reliable indicator of ischemia.

Clinical scenario

EKG Changes in Myocardial Infarction

"Can you tell me what is going on here?", Dr. Hicks asked the nursing student Eric by handing over a 12 lead EKG in his distinct Scottish accent. "oh oh!!, Eric is in trouble", Daniel who is the Telemetry nurse said with chuckles. Then Daniel continued, "I'm just kidding, looks like Dr. Hicks is in the mood to teach". "Yes, I am", Dr. Hicks replied by pulling his pager out of his pocket. He continued," excuse me, let me return this page". Dr. Hicks went on making the phone call. Once he finished, he turned around to Eric who was still looking at the EKG. "Did you find anything?", Dr. Hicks asked. Eric raised his head with hesitancy and said, "well, I'm not super familiar with these things. But I see some upside-down T waves in these areas". Eric said by pointing to V3, V4, V5 and V6 leads in the EKG. "Good observation", Dr. Hicks replied. "Yes, this guy has some T-wave inversion in the precordial leads. Do you know what it means?". "I'm not sure", Eric replied. "I think it is ischemia. That's what I vaguely remember from my class'". "Yes, that is correct", Dr. Hicks replied. "Myocardial ischemia and infarction cause different changes in the EKG. Do you know when the EKG worth million bucks?", Dr. Hicks asked. Eric nodded his head side to side. "This piece of paper is most valuable when someone is having MI. Getting a timely EKG and figuring out what exactly going on can make or break the case for saving lives. Have you heard of STEMI?" Dr. Hicks asked. "Yes, I do. Isn't that the sudden heart attack?" Eric replied. "Indeed, it is a heart

attack in progress and you only have hour to hour and a half to open the culprit vessel and save the myocardium. "Good, get a good EKG book and read it. It will help you all along your life. See you guys later", Dr Hicks said by getting up and walking towards the door.

EKG Changes in Myocardial Ischemia

- **Myocardial infarction in progress**
  Elevation of ST segment in leads corresponding to respective coronary artery territory. For example, in left anterior descending artery (LAD) occlusion, ST elevation is more pronounced in septal anterior leads, i.e. **V1- V4**.

- **Myocardial ischemia**
  Depression of ST segment with T wave inversion in ischemic territory.

- **Reciprocal changes**
  In an acute myocardial infarction, the area opposite of infarction shows reciprocal changes in ST segment. For example, in anterior wall myocardial infarction, ST segment elevation is seen in lead V1- V4. However, inferior leads (lead II, III and aVF) show ST segment depression.

Box 12.3 Characteristics of EKG in ischemia

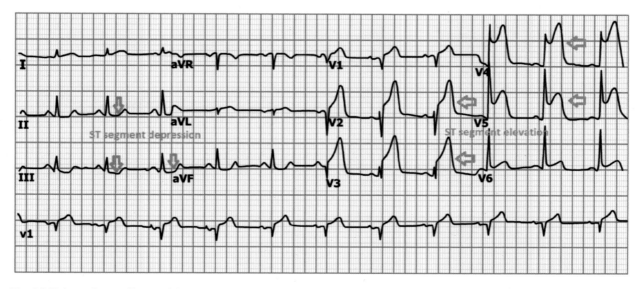

Fig 12.7 Anterior wall MI with its characteristic EKG changes (Note the presence of ST segment elevation in the anterior leads and ST segment depression in the inferior leads).

Prominent **Q wave** formation is an indication of **old myocardial infarction**. They are considered significant only when they are wide (**0.04 sec**) and larger (**greater than 1/3 of R wave**). Formation of Q wave takes more than 24 hours of myocardial ischemia. Therefore, *presence of Q wave in an EKG indicates that MI has happened more than 24 hours before.* This is a major determinant in selection of treatment options for individual patients.

Events Associated with Myocardial Infarction

- **Anterior MI:** This is the most lethal type of myocardial infarction due to the involvement of *left ventricle and septum.* If not intervened in a timely fashion, this pathologic process can markedly *reduce cardiac output* leading to dreadful consequences.

- **Inferior MI:** This produces *brady arrhythmias* and possible *heart block.* Since right coronary artery is the culprit vessel (artery that is occluded) and it supplies the right ventricle, patient may present with symptoms of fluid overload.

- **Posterior MI:** This is the most difficult type of myocardial infarction in terms of diagnosis. A regular surface EKG with precordial leads doesn't always show presence of a posterior MI. *Instead of normal QS wave pattern, presence of large R waves in V1 and V2 along with ST depression in antero-septal leads (V1- V4) represent posterior MI* (mirror image). It usually originates from a dominant posterior descending artery (PDA) or Circumflex coronary artery (LCx) that supplies posterior wall. Lead V7-V9, if taken, will show ST elevation.

Box 12.4 Clinical consequences of MI

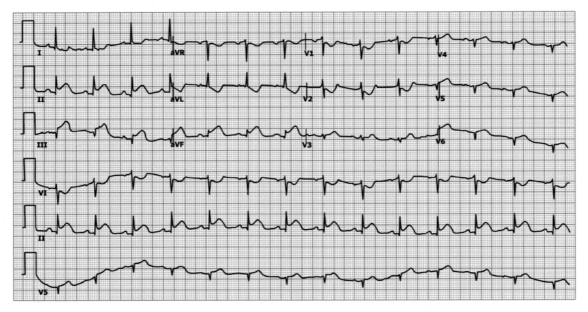

Fig 12.8 EKG findings in Inferior wall myocardial infarction. (Note the presence of ST segment elevation in the inferior leads (II, II and aVF) and mirror image changes in anterior leads (V1, V2)

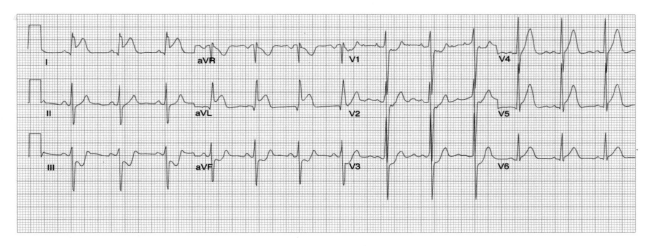

Fig 12.9 EKG in Lateral wall myocardial infarction. (Note the characteristic ST segment elevation in lateral leads (I, aVL) and mirror changes in the inferior leads (III and aVF).

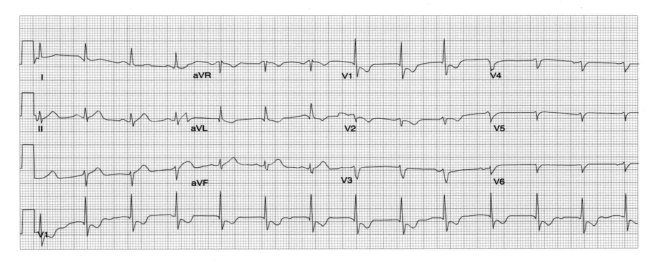

Fig 12.10 EKG tracing from Posterior wall myocardial infarction. (Note the presence of large R waves in Lead V1 with ST segment depression in V1 and V2).

Points to Remember!!!

- Atherosclerotic heart disease accounts for majority of myocardial ischemia and infarction.
- Stable angina pectoris is characterized by typical chest pain induced by physical or emotional exertion with characteristic nature and radiation, relieved by rest or sublingual nitroglycerin.

- Unstable angina has typical to atypical chest pain that may or may not respond to rest or sublingual nitroglycerin.
- Non-ST segment elevation myocardial infarction (NSTEMI) has characteristics of stable angina with elevated cardiac biomarkers and EKG changes.
- ST elevation myocardial infarction (STEMI) is caused by acute closure of

Treatment in Myocardial Infarction

Management of acute phase	Anti-ischemic treatment with • Oxygen • Nitroglycerin • Morphine • Aspirin • Beta-blockers
Preventing progression of acute phase	Anti-thrombolytic treatment with antiplatelets like • Clopidogrel • Prasugrel • Ticlopidine • Eptifibatide • Tirofiban • Abciximab • Heparin
Preventing of progression of risk factors	Risk factor reduction with • Statins and ACE inhibitors • Management of Diabetes, Smoking, life style etc.

Box 12.5 Treatment of myocardial infarction

Neurologic T wave

Acute ischemic stroke has sometimes a characteristic EKG finding with deep inverted T waves in multiple vascular distribution areas as follows.

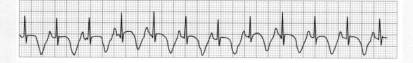

Fig 12.11 Classic deep T wave pattern in Acute stroke

Box 12.6 Neurologic T wave

a coronary artery leading to imminent myocardial injury.

- ST elevation MI has characteristic ST segment elevation in target leads depending on the artery affected.
- In anterior wall STEMI, lead V1 to V4 has ST elevations and inferior leads (lead II, III and aVF) have reciprocal changes in the form of ST segment depression.
- ST changes in isolated leads are not much of a diagnostic value.
- Major determinants of myocardial oxygen demand are heart rate, myocardial contractility and wall tension.

- Abnormal lipids, smoking, hypertension, diabetes mellitus etc. are common risk factors for development of coronary artery disease.
- In the event of myocardial ischemia lasts more than 20 min, permanent damage of myocardium called infarction may occur.
- Profound infarction of myocardial area especially that of left ventricle causes ischemic cardiomyopathy.
- Instead of ST segment elevation, myocardial ischemia causes depression of ST segment with T wave inversion in target leads.
- Presence of Q wave indicates myocardial infarction happened more than 24 hours prior to the presentation.
- Posterior wall myocardial infarction is one of the difficult diagnosis to be made from usual anterior chest wall EKG and is characterized by presence of large R waves in V1 and V2 in a regular EKG.
- Acute management of myocardial infarction depends on the type of MI.
- For STEMI, immediate and timely revascularization, either mechanical (PTCA with stents) or chemical (tPA or other thrombolytics) is of supreme priority.
- For NSTEMI or unstable angina, non-emergent revascularization along with risk factor modification is the treatment approach.

Test Your Understanding

1. Which of the following is not a characteristic of stable angina pectoris?
A   Chest pain induced by exertion
B   Chest pain relieved by nitroglycerin
C   Chest pain initiated without exertion
D   Squeezing substernal chest pain

2. Which of the following is a differentiating factor between stable angina and non-ST segment elevation myocardial infarction?
A   Typical chest pain with radiation
B   Relieved by rest or sublingual nitroglycerin
C   Absence of cardiac enzymes elevation
D   Presence of elevated troponin or CKMB

3. Which of the following EKG finding is consistent with inferior wall myocardial infarction?
A   ST depression in lead II and III
B   Elevation of ST segment in lead aVL, V5 and V6
C   ST segment elevation in lead II, III and aVF
D   Presence of large T wave in V6

4. Which of the following is not a finding in anterior wall ST elevation MI?
A   ST segment elevation in lead V3 and V4
B   ST segment depression in lead II and aVF
C   ST segment elevation in lead II and III
D   T wave inversion in lead III and aVF

5. Coronary atherosclerosis risk factors include all of the following except_____?
A   Increased HDL cholesterol
B   Increased LDL cholesterol
C   Smoking
D   Diabetes mellitus

6. Which of the following finding is not seen in lateral wall myocardial infarction?
A   ST elevation in III and aVF

B   ST elevation in aVL and V5

C   ST elevation in V5 and V6

D   ST elevation in lead I, V5 and V6

7. One of the serious complications of anterior wall MI is _____?

A   Right ventricular hypertrophy

B   Left ventricular dysfunction

C   Right atrial dysfunction

D   Bradycardia

8. Which of the following is not a treatment option for non-ST segment elevation myocardial infarction?

A   PTCA and stent

B   Use of tPA

C   Use of aspirin and nitroglycerin

D   Use of beta-blockers

Answers

1.   C   Chest pain initiated without exertion

2.   D   Presence of elevated troponin or CKMB

3.   C   ST segment elevation in lead II, III and aVF

4.   C   ST segment elevation in lead II and III

5.   A   Increased HDL cholesterol

6.   A   ST elevation in III and aVF

7.   B   Left ventricular dysfunction

8.   B   Use of tPA

CHAPTER 13

General Diagnostic Value of EKG

In this chapter

- Right atrial overload
- Left atrial overload
- Right ventricular hypertrophy
- Cor-pulmonale due to COPD
- Left ventricular hypertrophy
- Pulmonary embolus

Clinical scenario

"This EKG looks strange", Diana said to Sherry by pointing to the tall QRS complex in the 12 lead EKG in her hand. Diana, who is a student nurse doing clinical rotation with one of the senior step-down unit nurse Sherry, continued, "these QRS complexes are so tall. Why is that?". "Let me see", sherry said and continued, "this is LVH. Do you know what it is?". Diana nodded her head and said, "I heard about it somewhere. But honest with you, I don't know". "Well… LVH causes thickness of the left ventricular wall. Hypertrophy means increase in size of the cells. Due to various reasons, the heart muscle around the left ventricle start growing in size, end up in a thick ventricular wall. When it happened to the left ventricle, it is called left ventricular hypertrophy". Sherry said. "When there is lot of muscle, there is a big electrical wave in the EKG", Sherry continued. "Is it the thickness of the left ventricle the only

thing shows up in the EKG?" Diana asked. "No, no. There are all kinds of stuff that make changes in EKG... like enlargement of chambers especially atrium, change in electrolytes like potassium, pulmonary embolism and so on."

Structural changes in chambers of the heart create substantial electrocardiographic evidence as it changes the duration and force of electrical activity within the myocardium. Looking at specific leads that are designated for monitoring individual areas of the heart, a 12 lead EKG may provide initial clues for underlying pathophysiologic process. Mostly, enlargement or thickening of chambers produce *wide or tall waveforms* in corresponding leads.

Left Atrial Enlargement

In a normal heart, the sequence of atrial activation starts from right atrium (since SA node is situated here), which then followed by the left atrium because of the minute travelling delay for impulse from right to left chamber. This delayed activation of the left atrium leads to a *slight notching of P wave*. Hypertrophy or scarring of the atrial wall resulting from left atrial enlargement increases this Inter atrial delay. Similar to any other conduction delay, the impulses from right atrium takes longer to depolarize the enlarged left atrium, leading to wide P wave (>0.12 sec) with a pronounced notching. This increase in duration of P wave is known as classic '*P mitrale*' sign. These changes are evident in the inferior leads such as lead **III** and **aVF**. In the anterior precordial lead **V1**, left atrial enlargement may produce a deeply inverted P wave.

Right Atrial Hypertrophy

Similar to the mechanism seen in the left atrial enlargement, scarring and hypertrophy of right atrium causes *delay in depolarization of right atrium*. Therefore, both atria will depolarize *simultaneously rather than sequentially* creating a *narrow and tall P wave* called '*P Pulmonale*'. This change is pronounced in lead **II** and **V1**. In severe right atrial enlargement, the right atrium may become so large that it extent towards the left atrium creating an inverted P wave in lead **V1** mimicking EKG change of left atrial enlargement.

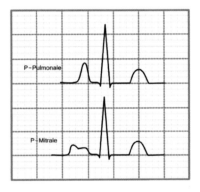

Fig 13.1 Wide and notched P wave in LA enlargement

EKG Criteria for Atrial Enlargement

Right Atrial Hypertrophy
- Narrow and tall **P** wave (*P Pulmonale*) in Lead **II** and **V1**

Left Atrial Hypertrophy
- Wide and notched **P** wave (>0.12 Sec) in lead **III** and **aVF** (*P Mitrale*)
- Deep inverted **P** wave in **V1**

Box 13.1 EKG criteria for atrial hypertrophy

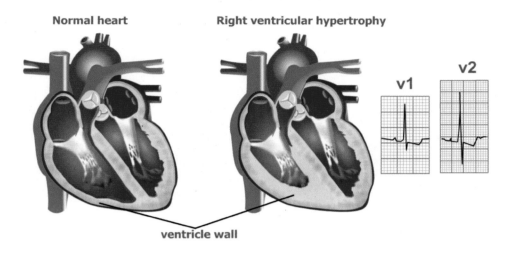

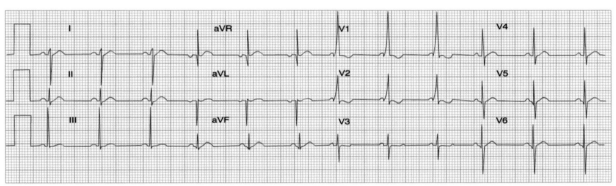

Fig 13.2 Tall R wave in VI and V2- a sign of right ventricular hypertrophy

Right Ventricular Hypertrophy

Hypertrophy of right ventricle (RVH) is seen in clinical conditions such as *advanced COPD*, *corpulmonale*, *tricuspid* or *pulmonic stenosis* and as a sequel of *mitral stenosis (due to back flow of blood from left atrium through pulmonary circulation)*. Right ventricular wall thickness increases to compensate for elevated right ventricular pressure caused by any of these underlying disease conditions. This increased muscle mass causes *tall R waves* in *anterior precordial* leads (*lead V1 and V2*) and *deep S waves* in *lead V5 and V6*.

Unlike normal 12 lead EKG, right ventricular hypertrophy (RVH) causes *tall R waves and small S waves* in *lead V1* and *V2* creating an **R: S ratio >1**. However, before jumping into the conclusion of relatively less acute right ventricular hypertrophy, we have to exclude other more serious causes of increased R: S ratio such as *posterior wall myocardial infarction*, *WPW syndrome*, *hypertrophic cardiomyopathy* etc. In some patients, this reversal of R: S ratio can be a normal variant without any underlying pathology. Excessive thickening of ventricular wall may cause sub endocardial ischemia in the right ventricular wall, leading to ST segment and T wave changes in the right-sided precordial leads. Right ventricular hypertrophy is also associated with *right axis deviation*.

EKG Criteria for Right Ventricular Hypertrophy

- Right axis deviation
- Tall **R** waves in **V1** and **V2** (increased R: S ratio)
- Deep **S** waves in **V5** and **V6**
- ST or T wave abnormalities (*strain pattern*) in the inferior leads
- Signs of right atrial hypertrophy (**P pulmonale**)

Box 13.2 EKG criteria for Right Ventricular hypertrophy (RVH)

Left Ventricular Hypertrophy

Being the main pumping chamber of the heart, left ventricle has to increase its effort in any event that causes obstruction of blood flow into the systemic circulation. Common causes that increase workload of the left ventricle are *aortic stenosis*, *hypertrophic cardiomyopathy*, *long-standing elevated blood pressure* etc. The constant strain imparted on the left ventricle results in *increasing muscle mass* and *subsequent thickening* of the ventricular wall in order to assist in effective contraction. The thickened ventricular wall creates more resistance for electrical impulse to travel, leading to *slightly wide QRS complexes*.

At the same time, increased muscle mass causes *elevated amplitude* of resulting waveform. There may be *left axis deviation* because of the increased muscle mass in the left ventricle. Similar to the right ventricular hypertrophy, sub endocardial ischemic changes create down sloping ST segment and inverted T wave (*strain pattern*) in left lateral leads (lead **I**, **aVL**, **V5** and **V6**).

There are multiple EKG criteria used to diagnose left ventricular hypertrophy (LVH) from a 12 lead EKG. Most common and reliable criteria are shown in the table.

EKG Criteria for Left Ventricular Hypertrophy

Sokolow and Lyon Index

- Amplitude of **S** wave in lead **V1** and **R** wave in lead **V5** or **V6** greater than or equal to 35mm

$$S\ V1 + R\ V5/V6 >= 35mm$$
$$R\ in\ aVL >=11\ mm$$

Cornell Criteria

- Amplitude of **R** wave in **aVL** and **S** wave in **V3** greater than 28 mm in men or greater than 20 mm in women

$$R\ aVL + S\ V3 > 28 - men$$
$$> 20 - women$$

Box 13.3 EKG criteria for LVH

Bi-ventricular Hypertrophy

In patients with advanced stages of underlying diseases, coexistence of both right and left ventricular hypertrophy is not uncommon. These patients may have EKG satisfying voltage

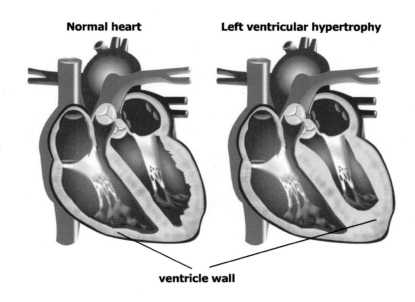

Normal heart   **Left ventricular hypertrophy**

ventricle wall

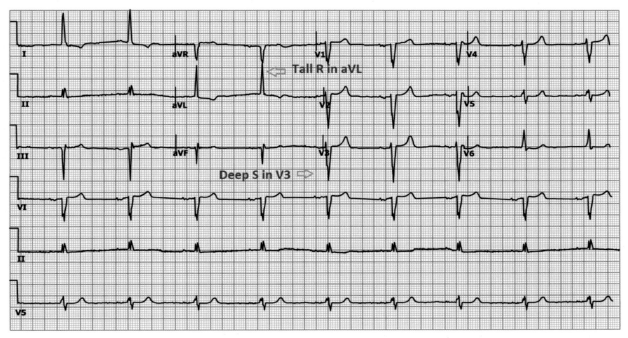

Fig 13.3 left ventricular hypertrophy (Note the presence of tall R waves in Lead III and deep S waves in V3 suggesting LVH)

criteria for *LVH in the precordial leads* along with *right axis deviation in limb leads* or *tall R waves in precordial V1 and V2*. Some of them also have coexisting left atrial enlargement with the characteristic wide P wave as discussed earlier. Biventricular hypertrophy is also seen in children with ventricular septal defect. These children have EKG showing tall biphasic R waves in precordial leads known as Katz-Wachtel phenomena as shown in the picture.

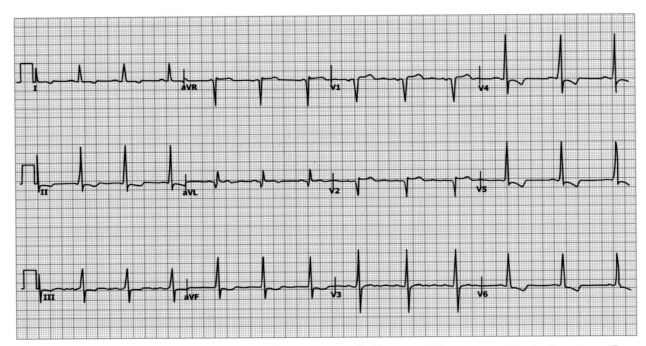

Fig 13.4 Left Ventricular Hypertrophy (Note the presence of tall precordial R waves with strain pattern. Even though this EKG doesn't meet above-mentioned criteria for LVH, this patient had echocardiogram findings confirming left ventricular hypertrophy).

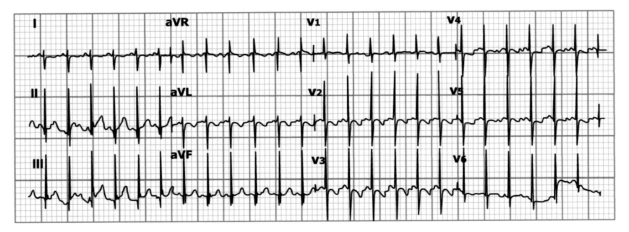

Fig 13.5 Biventricular hypertrophy (Note the presence of tall precordial biphasic R waves with right axis deviation (Negative Lead I and positive aVF) and prominent R waves in V1).

Pulmonary Embolism

Even though not universally present, many patients with massive acute pulmonary embolism shows characteristic EKG changes such as a *prominent S wave in lead I*, *presence of Q wave* and *inverted T wave in lead III* (**S1Q3T3 pattern**), *ST segment and T wave changes in anterior precordial leads* (right ventricular strain pattern), new *incomplete right bundle branch block* and *sinus tachycardia* (Fig 13.6).

Pericarditis

Pericarditis and acute pericardial effusion can create characteristic EKG changes that mimic signs of acute STEMI due to the inflammation of epicardium. There may also be typical *PR segment depression*. Here, both ST and PR segments deviate in opposite direction. In pericarditis, due to more generalized inflammation and resulting tissue injury compared to focused STEMI, *ST segment elevation may be wide spread in varying degrees in multiple leads* than focused leads (Fig 13.7).

Pericardial Effusion or Cardiac Tamponade

Pericardial effusion or cardiac tamponade can develop from acute or chronic collection of fluid within the pericardium. Acute pericarditis can be a reason for pericardial effusion or cardiac tamponade. In this situation, because of the presence of fluid outside the heart, surface EKG will show *low amplitude or low voltage complexes*. These could also be presence of *alteration in amplitude of QRS in adjacent beats* called **electrical alternans** as shown in Fig 13.8.

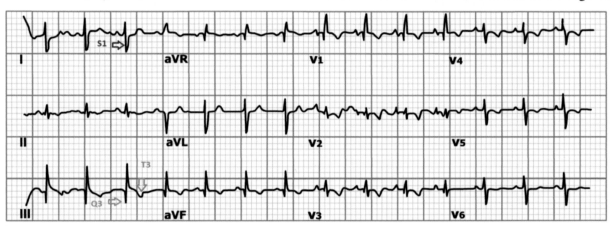

Fig 13.6 Pulmonary embolism (Even though the patient doesn't have tachycardia, this EKG has prominent S in lead I, Q and inverted T waves in lead III along with incomplete RBBB and inverted T waves in anterior precordial leads (V1-V3) suggesting right ventricular strain pattern.

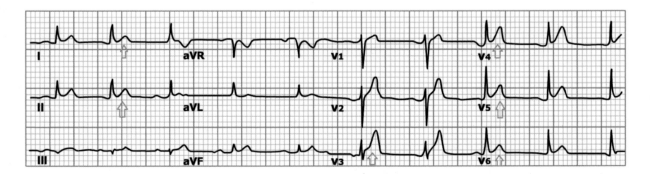

Fig 13.7 Acute pericarditis (Note the presence of diffuse ST segment elevation in inferior, lateral and anterior leads denoting possible wide spread inflammation).

EKG Findings in Electrolyte Imbalance

Since electrolytes like Potassium, Calcium and Magnesium play a vital role in various electrical and contractile functions of the heart, any change in the availability of these elements can produce characteristic changes in the resulting EKG as shown in the Box 13.3.

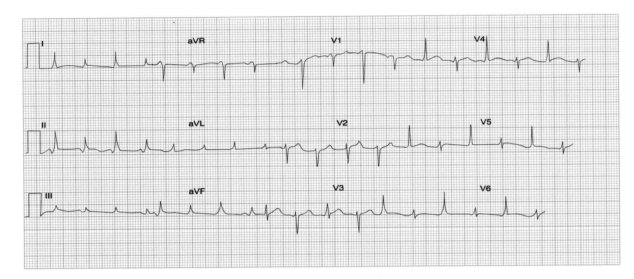

Fig 13.8 Electrical alternans (Note the presence of varying amplitude of QRS from beat to beat).

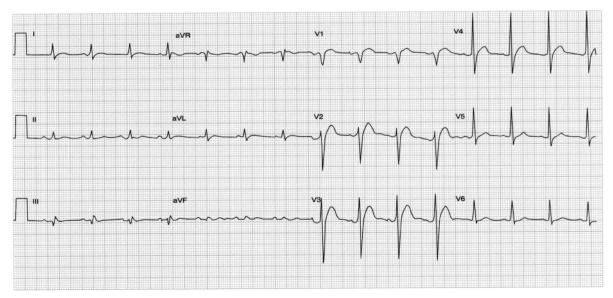

Fig 13.9 EKG changes in hypercalcemia

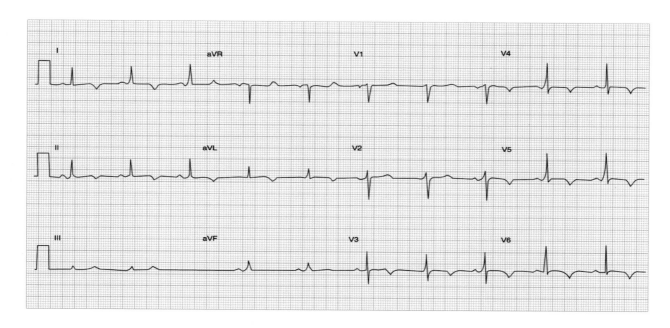

Fig 13.10 Hypocalcemia (Note the presence of long ST segment without increase in duration of T wave).

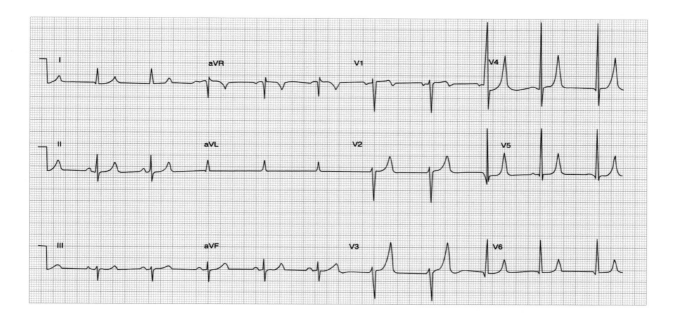

Fig 13.11 Hyperkalemia (Note the presence of tall peaked T waves with narrow base in the precordial leads).

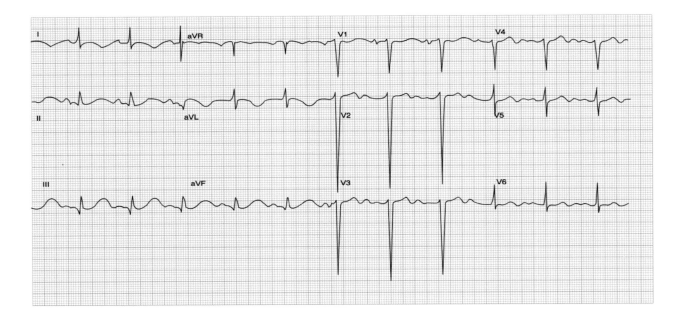

Fig 13.12 Hypokalemia (Note the presence of dominant U waves in precordial leads).

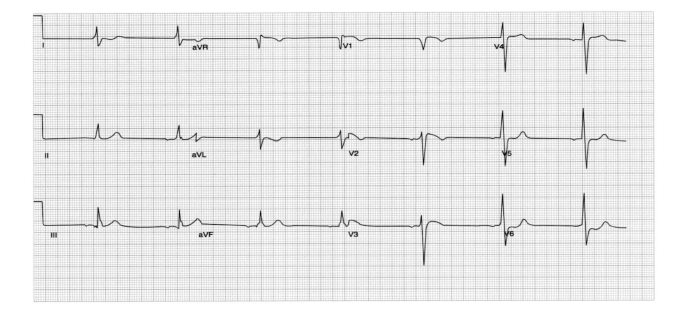

Fig 13.13 Hypernatremia (Note the presence of 'Brugada like' pattern).

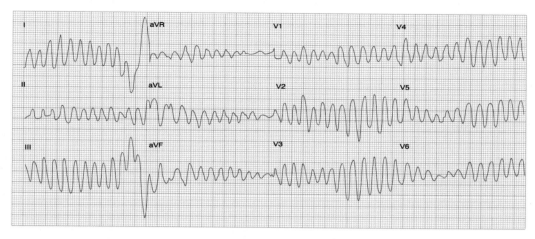

Fig 13.14 Hypomagnesemia showing as polymorphic VT (Torsades).

Effects of Electrolyte Imbalance in 12 lead EKG

Ion	Hypo-	Hyper-
Calcium	• Prolonged QTc • Flat or inverted T waves • Prolonged ST segments without increased duration of T waves	• Short QTc • PR segment prolongation

Potassium	• Tall U waves
	• Small T waves
	• Large P waves
	• ST depression
		5.5 - 7.5 mEq/L
		  • Tall peaked T waves
		  • Reversible LAFB or LPFB
		7.5 - 10.0 mEq/L
		  • First degree AV block
		  • Flat/ wide/absent P wave
		  • ST segment depression
		  • Significant bradycardia
		> 10.0 mEq/L
		  • LBBB, RBBB or IVCD
		  • V tach /V fib
		  • Idioventricular rhythm

Sodium	• 'Brugada' like appearance (ST elevation in V1 -V3 with RBBB)	
Magnesium	• Peak T waves • Prominent U waves • Prolong QRS • ST depression • Ventricular arrhythmia including Torsades de Pointes	• Prolonged PR interval • Increased QRS duration • Increased QT interval • Complete heart block • Cardiac arrest if Mg > 15 mEq/L

LAFB- Left anterior fascicular block; LPFB- left Posterior fascicular block; IVCD- interventricular conduction delay

Box 13.4 Effect of electrolyte imbalance in EKG

Points to Remember!!!

- Left atrial enlargement produces slightly notched P wave that is more pronounced in lead III and aVF, called p mitrale sign.
- Instead of the notched P wave as in the left atrial enlargement, right atrial hypertrophy EKG has a narrow and tall P wave called P Pulmonale.
- Because of the increased muscle mass in the right ventricle during right ventricular hypertrophy, there are tall R waves in lead V1 and V2 and deep S waves in V5 and V6.
- Right ventricular hypertrophy should be differentiated from that of posterior wall of MI, WPW syndrome, hypertrophic cardiomyopathy etc.
- Right ventricular hypertrophy also causes right axis deviation.
- Left ventricular hypertrophy is caused by aortic stenosis, hypertrophic cardiomyopathy, long-standing elevated blood pressure etc.
- Because of the increased muscle mass, tall R waves are seen in the lateral and precordial leads.
- Along with tall R waves, down sloping ST segment and inverted T waves (strain pattern) are also seen in LVH.
- Most reliable and widely accepted criteria for left ventricular hypertrophy is Cornell criteria where R aVL + S V3 > 28 mm in men/> 20 mm in women.
- Pulmonary embolism generates prominent S wave in lead I, presence of Q and inverted T wave in lead III (S1 Q3 T3).
- Pericarditis produces EKG similar to that of a STEMI; however, with varying degrees of generalized ST elevation.

Test Your Understanding

1. 12 lead EKG of a patient with left atrial enlargement involve_____?
A   Tall and narrow R waves
B   Tall and wide R waves
C   Tall and narrow P wave
D   Notched P wave

2. Which of the following is a characteristic EKG finding in right ventricular hypertrophy?
A   Deep S waves in lead V1 and V2
B   Deep S waves in V5 and V6
C   Tall R wave in V5 and V6
D   Inverted P wave in lead I

3. Which of the following is one of the possible differential diagnoses for an EKG with R waves in lead V1 and V2?
A   Right atrial enlargement
B   Left atrial enlargement
C   Posterior wall MI
D   Left ventricular hypertrophy

4. Which of the following is a possible causative factor for left ventricular hypertrophy?
A   Dilated cardiomyopathy
B   Long-standing hypotension
C   Tricuspid regurgitation
D   Aortic stenosis

5. Which of the following is a characteristic EKG finding in acute pulmonary embolism?
A   Sinus bradycardia
B   Ventricular fibrillation
C   Prominent S in lead I with presence of Q and T inversion in lead III
D   Left bundle branch block

Answers

1. D   Notched P wave
2. B   Deep S waves in V5 and V6
3. C   Posterior wall MI
4. D   Aortic stenosis
5. C   Prominent S in lead I with presence of Q and T inversion in lead III

CHAPTER 14

Cardiac Pharmacology

In this chapter

- Antiarrhythmics – classification
- Class I Antiarrhythmics
- Class II Antiarrhythmics
- Class III Antiarrhythmics
- Class IV Antiarrhythmics

Clinical scenario

"Tell me again, what is this patient here for?" Tina asked Brenda during the shift report in the telemetry unit. Tina is a travel nurse, working at this unit for the first time. "Like I said, Mr. Carter is here for monitoring while initiating Flecainide", Brenda replied. "Hum... I never heard of that drug, what is it for?" Tina asked. "It is a class 1 antiarrhythmic agent. More precisely, it is a class IC agent used for treatment of atrial fibrillation. We have our electrophysiologist, Dr. Hansen uses this drug in many patients. Even though they treat arrhythmia, they can cause arrhythmia by themselves. Flecainide and Propafenone are the 2 drugs which belong to Class 1C antiarrhythmic agents. Since they can cause arrhythmia, patients who started on these drugs should be monitored for 48 to 72 hours in the hospital. Believe me, Mr. Carter is going to be your best patient for the entire shift. He is a very pleasant

gentleman who rarely calls you for anything. He just walks around and do his thing. I know he is bored. Last night he was out here at the nurse's station and joking with all of us. He is our captive for another 48 hours", Brenda replied. "Oh, okay. That's good. At least I'll have one easy patient with 2 difficult ones", Tina said. "Well, you don't want to completely ignore this patient. Dr. Hansen is very particular about his patients. He expects us nurses to be in charge and report to him any events. I would definitely get a 12 lead this morning and report him if there are any events", Brenda replied. "Okay, I can do that". Tina said. "Let's go and see Mr. Carter. I'll introduce you to him", Brenda said.

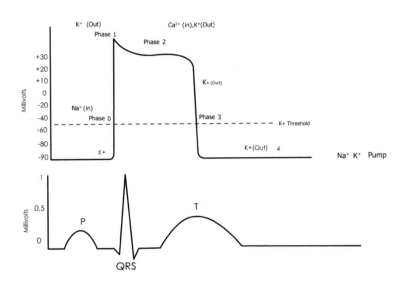

Fig 14.1 Cardiac action potential curve

From the information what we discussed in earlier chapters, it is evident that contractile function of myocardium is a complex process involving electrical, chemical and mechanical components at various levels. To the very basis of this process resides movement of ions such as calcium, sodium and potassium. Even though there are other trace elements involved in the overall process, these ions are of particularly important because of the way many of our cardiac medications work in the system.

Antiarrhythmic Drugs

These medications are used for management of heart rhythm disorders and are classified into different groups based on their pharmacodynamics. The most common and widely accepted classification is known as Vaughan Williams classification. Here, antiarrhythmic agents are grouped based on the action at various levels of cardiac action potential curve. All of these agents essentially regulate flow of ions to and from the myocytes and thereby manipulate either normal or abnormal conduction pathways.

Based on the electrical ions they regulate; antiarrhythmic drugs are classified largely into four groups. Class **I** agents are sodium channel blockers, beta-blockers in class **II**, potassium channel blockers in class **III** and calcium channel blockers in class IV. Adenosine and digoxin are classified as class **V** in the system. Even though there are other classifications available that are more complex, Vaughan Williams classification provides a bird's eye view on antiarrhythmic drugs and provide easier understanding based on its relationship with *cardiac action potential curve*. Even though each drug is categorized in a specific group, their effects may overlap each other. In general, *sodium channel blockers slow down the conduction velocity whereas, potassium channel blockers decrease excitability*.

Class I Antiarrhythmics

These agents are otherwise called sodium channel blockers that control *movement of sodium ions in phase 0* of cardiac action potential curve. By modulating sodium ions at this stage, these drugs can essentially influence the onset of cardiac action potential. Depending on the ease of binding and dissociation with the receptor sites, they are further classified into class **1C** (having *slowest rate of binding and dissociation*), class **1A** (with *intermediate binding and dissociation*) and class **1B** (has *rapid binding and release*). As these agents vary in their rate of receptor attachment, it is of great use in managing both faster and slower rhythms. For example, class 1C drugs (**Flecainide** and **Propafenone**) when used during faster heart rate takes *more time to*

Classification of Antiarrhythmic Drugs

Class	Type	Drugs
Class I A	Sodium channel blockers	• Procainamide • Quinidine • Disopyramide
Class IB		• Lidocaine • Mexiletine
Class IC		• Flecainide • Propafenone
Class II	Beta blockers	• Carvedilol • Metoprolol
Class III	Potassium channel blockers	• Amiodarone • Sotalol • Dronedarone • Ibutilide • Dofetilide
Class IV	Calcium channel blockers	• Verapamil • Diltiazem
Class V		• Digoxin • Adenosine • Magnesium sulphate

Box 14.1 Classification of antiarrhythmic drugs

dissociate from the receptor sites and make less number of receptors available for active contractile function. This effect essentially lowers the heart rate because of the lack of resources to continue rapid action potential cycles. This property is called use dependent channel block. They primarily block sodium channels open for business and thereby slow down conduction. However, these agents may produce pro arrhythmic activity in the myocardium with underlying injury. Therefore, these agents are *not indicated* in patients with *structural heart disease.* The efficacy of sodium channel blocking property is *highest for class 1C drugs, followed by class 1A and class 1B.*

Class 1A

Sodium channel blocking properties of these agents are *intermediate* to that of other catagories of class I antiarrhythmic drugs. Quinidine, Procainamide and Disopyramide are prime examples of this group. Among these, Quinidine has many drug-to-drug interactions especially when using with Verapamil, Phenytoin, digoxin etc. Pro-arrhythmic effect of these medications can cause formation of Torsades De Pointes especially in patients with prolonged base line QT interval and electrolyte abnormalities. If the baseline *QTC is greater than 500 ms*, use of antiarrhythmics should be *cautioned.* For susceptible patients, initiation of these drugs requires *in hospital monitoring.* Quinidine is used for treatment of ventricular arrhythmias and Procainamide for atrial fibrillation.

Class 1B

Lidocaine and Mexiletine are classified into class **1B** antiarrhythmics. They are particularly *useful in treating ventricular arrhythmias* in the setting of myocardial infarction because

of their efficacy in *fast heart rate and in abnormal myocardium.* Lidocaine has extensive first pass metabolism in the liver that essentially reduces availability of drug when taken orally and therefore needs to be administered intravenously. Mexiletine is used as an *oral equivalent* of Lidocaine in many situations. Compared to that of Lidocaine, Mexiletine has minimal hemodynamic side effects. *Nystagmus* is a common early indication of Lidocaine toxicity.

Class 1C

Flecainide and Propafenone are used for treatment of *atrial fibrillation.* In patients *with structural heart disease* such as prior history of myocardium ischemia and infarction, Flecainide and Propafenone can cause harmful effects and therefore are *contraindicated.*

Class II Antiarrhythmics

These agents are otherwise known as beta-blockers, with their characteristic beta-adrenergic receptor blockade property. Depending on the lipid solubility, their plasma half-life differs. For example, lipid soluble beta-blockers such as Metoprolol and Propranolol metabolize through liver and have shorter half-life however, Atenolol that has prominent renal clearance stays in the blood longer. Beta-blockers can be broadly classified in to selective beta I receptor blockers (cardio selective) or non-selective beta blockers (non-cardio selective). Since beta-2 receptors are seen in vascular, smooth muscle and myocardial cells, *non-selective beta-blockers have global effect* on these target areas. Since *beta-1 receptor blockers selectively influence the heart,* they are of great use in clinical situations such as bronchial asthma where beta-2 receptors can cause adverse effects.

In terms of pharmacodynamics of beta-blockers, they counteract the effect of catecholamine at beta-adrenergic receptor sites. This results in *decreasing contractility* (*negative inotropic effect*) and slowing of the heart rate by *reducing automaticity* (*negative chronotropic effect*). These agents are useful in treating both ventricular and atrial arrhythmia especially during high catecholamine states like myocardial ischemia and perioperative stage. Sotalol, even though a beta-blocker, has more class **III** antiarrhythmic properties. Examples of beta-blockers are shown in the box.

Classification of Beta-Blockers

Non-selective	• Propranolol
	• Timolol
	• Labetalol
	• Carvedilol
	• Sotalol*
	• Pindolol
	• Bucindolol
Beta -2 Selective	• Metoprolol
	• Atenolol
	• Bisoprolol
	• Esmolol
	• Betaxolo

* Has more class III antiarrhythmic property

Box 14.2 Classification of beta-blockers

Beta-blockers have a wide range of therapeutic usage extending from treatment of stage fright to effective management of supraventricular and ventricular arrhythmias. They are also useful in management of hypertension, congestive heart failure, angina pectoris, hypertrophic obstructive cardiomyopathy, mitral valve prolapse etc.

Clinical scenario

"Can you please start Amiodarone drip? This guy seems to be in Afib RVR", Dr. Bennett asked ICU nurse Jim. "Sure, you want me to bolus him. Right?" "Yes please, then start the drip per protocol", Dr. Bennett replied. "Got it, I'm on it. Let's go to the med room, my friend". Jim said to Danny who is a student nurse working with him today as he got up from the nurses' station. Jim and Danny started amiodarone for the patient. Later that day Danny asked Jim. "So, this morning Dr. Benson asked us to give amiodarone for Mrs. Bush and room 12. Was it for lowering her heart rate?". "Yes, that was one of the objective", Jim continued. "You know, amiodarone is an antiarrhythmic drug. We can use amiodarone for many different types of arrhythmia. One of the common one is atrial fibrillation. You know about cardioversion, right?" "Isn't it the electric shocking of the heart?" Danny asked. "Yes, that is one form of cardioversion. When we use electricity, it is called electrical cardioversion. Amiodarone is a medicine that you can use for chemical cardioversion. It can convert arrhythmias to normal sinus rhythm or control the rate when it is too fast. The only problem is that amiodarone sits around in the body for a while. Half-life of amiodarone in the

body is around 58 days", Jim replied. "Wow, that is interesting". Danny said. "Yup, if you use it for long-term, amiodarone can cause a lot of side effects. But it is a great drug for acute control of arrhythmia."

Class III Antiarrhythmics

This group of medications have characteristic *potassium channel blocking* properties. Exceptions are Sotalol, which has *both beta blocking and potassium channel blocking* properties and Amiodarone that has a wide range of properties extending from *class 1 to 4 effects*. These medications are particularly useful in atrial fibrillation, flutter and ventricular tachyarrhythmia. They cause *increase in duration of cardiac action potential* and therefore *prolong QT interval* in EKG.

Amiodarone is a major player among class III antiarrhythmic drugs and has a wide range of use in both emergent and chronic situations. When given intravenously during an *acute myocardial event, Amiodarone* shows more of *class I* and *IV properties* (*sodium* and *calcium channel blocking*) and thereby effectively *treats faster ventricular arrhythmias*. It is highly fat-soluble and takes many weeks before reaching steady state in the body. Because of this extensive fat solubility and distribution, Amiodarone is *not dialyzable,* and it stays in body for longer duration. Amiodarone is predominantly *metabolized through liver*. Unlike many other antiarrhythmic drugs such as Sotalol, Procainamide etc., Amiodarone *does not require hospitalization* for initiation because of its low propensity for producing polymorphic VT compared to other agents.

There are many side effects of Amiodarone, mostly from chronic use including chronic interstitial pneumonitis, thyroid dysfunction, photosensitivity, peripheral neuropathy etc. Like many other antiarrhythmics, Amiodarone also has pro-arrhythmic effect due to *Q-T prolongation*. It can also cause bradycardia especially with concomitant use of beta-blockers. Amiodarone has also shown to increase defibrillation threshold (energy required for successful conversion of ventricular tachyarrhythmia) in chronic use. Amiodarone has interaction with Digoxin and Coumadin and therefore requires careful *monitoring and dose adjustments*.

Sotalol, having both beta blocking and potassium channel blocking properties is widely used for management of *atrial fibrillation* especially in patients *with implantable defibrillator*. Unlike Amiodarone, *Sotalol reduces the fibrillation threshold*. Side effects of Sotalol include *bradycardia* that is due to beta blocking property and *Q-T prolongation* and *risk of polymorphic VT* (Torsades) as part of potassium channel blocking. Because of predominant renal clearance, Sotalol is *not ideal in renal dysfunction*. In patients with risk factors for polymorphic VT (Torsades), initiation of Sotalol should only be done under monitoring in the hospital.

Class IV Antiarrhythmics

These agents are otherwise known as Calcium channel blockers. Depending on the chemical properties and resulting pharmacodynamic effect, calcium channel blockers are classified into Dihydropyridine (Nifedipine, Amlodipine, Felodipine, Nicardipine etc.) and non-dihydropyridine (Verapamil and Diltiazem). Because of the predominant inhibitory effect on the SA and the AV node, *non-dihydropyridine calcium channel blockers have pertinent electrophysiologic properties* compared to that of dihydropyridines. Therefore, Verapamil and Diltiazem are commonly used for *rate control* especially in atrial arrhythmias. These agents *prolong AV node conduction* and *refractoriness* and thereby reduce ventricular rate in AV nodal re-entry tachycardia. They do not have much effect on ventricular arrhythmias. Non-dihydropyridine calcium channel blockers are used for various other purposes in cardiovascular medicine including management of hypertension, vasospastic angina, hypertrophic cardiomyopathy etc.

Calcium channel blockers can cause *bradycardia* and especially orthostatic *hypotension*. These agents are *not indicated in pregnancy, post myocardial infarction, severe sinus node dysfunction* or *conduction disturbance, WPW syndrome, severe aortic stenosis* etc. In the event of digoxin toxicity, concomitant use of Verapamil can cause complete heart block. Overdose with calcium channel blockers can be treated with administration of calcium gluconate.

Class V Antiarrhythmics

Digoxin and Adenosine are categorized in this group. Among these, Digoxin implies its antiarrhythmic properties due to *increased vagal tone*. It produces *increasing contractility* (*positive inotropic effect*) in myocardium by *increasing intracellular calcium* concentration. Because of the smaller therapeutic window (**0.8 - 1.2** ng/ml), Digoxin needs *frequent monitoring of blood levels*. It also has interaction with many other drugs including Amiodarone, warfarin etc. In toxic dosage, digoxin causes *high-grade atrioventricular block* or *accelerated junctional rhythm* and at times *ventricular tachycardia*.

Effect of Digoxin in EKG

Digitalis effect

- Short QT interval
- Down sloping ST depression ('Reverse tick mark' appearance as shown in Lead V5, V6 in Fig 14.2)
- decreased T wave amplitude
- Long PR interval

Digoxin Toxicity

- Any type of arrhythmia resulting from either a disturbance in impulse formation or conduction except Bundle branch block like
  - Paroxysmal atrial tachycardia,
  - Atrial fibrillation with heart block
  - Second or third-degree heart block
  - Accelerated junctional or Idioventricular rhythm

Box 14.3 Effect of Digitalis in EKG

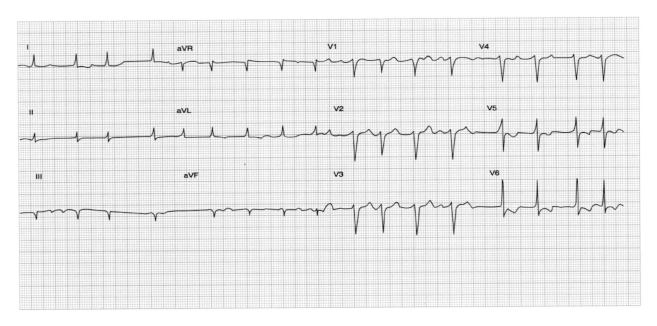

Fig 14.2 Digitalis effect (Note the presence of 'reverse tick mark' appearance of ST segment in Lead V5 and V6).

In patients with **WPW pattern** of EKG, digoxin administration should be avoided because of the risk of *delaying AV nodal conduction and promoting accessory pathway*, leading to *ventricular tachyarrhythmia*. **Digoxin immune FAB** antibody therapy can be used in severe digoxin toxicity. Tachyarrhythmia secondary to digoxin toxicity should not be treated with DC cardioversion because of the risk of ventricular tachycardia.

Adenosine acts through specialized *potassium channels* within the atrium, SA and AV node. Because of the lack of these channels in ventricular myocardium, Adenosine *doesn't have any direct effect on ventricles*. Adenosine has a very short half-life. Rapid intravenous injection of adenosine produces profound and transient AV nodal conduction block and therefore useful in termination of **paroxysmal SVT**. If the patient has concomitant use of **Theophylline**, *Adenosine does not work* because of the adenosine receptor blockade from Theophylline. Because of the possible micro re-entry circuit within atria, Adenosine can produce *atrial fibrillation in 10-15% of patients*. Use of **Dipyridamole** can prolong the effect of adenosine and therefore should be use with caution.

Points to Remember!!!

- Antiarrhythmic drugs are classified based on their mechanism of action into class I (sodium channel blockers), class II (beta-blockers), class III (potassium channel blockers) and class IV (calcium channel blockers).

- Class I antiarrhythmic are further classified into class 1A (Quinidine, Procainamide and Disopyramide), class 1B (Lidocaine and Mexiletine) and class 1C (Flecainide and Propafenone).

- Class I antiarrhythmic drugs work on phase 0 of myocardial action potential curve.

- Among class I antiarrhythmics, class 1C drugs have maximum sodium channel blocking property.

- Class I drugs can prolong QT interval and therefore needs to be monitored in the hospital on initiation.
- Lidocaine and Mexiletine are classified into class 1B antiarrhythmics, particularly useful in treating ventricular arrhythmias in the event of myocardial infarction.
- Flecainide and Propafenone are major class 1C antiarrhythmics, used for treatment of atrial fibrillation and are contraindicated in structural heart disease.
- Beta-blockers constitute class II antiarrhythmics.
- Beta-blockers can be cardio selective and non-selective depending on specificity to beta-1 or beta-2 receptors.
- Beta-blockers cause negative inotropic effect (reduce contractility) and negative chronotropic effect (reduce automaticity).
- Class III antiarrhythmic drugs are otherwise known as potassium channel blockers.
- Sotalol has both beta blocking and potassium channel blocking activity.
- Amiodarone has predominant class III antiarrhythmic property; however, has class 1 to 4 effect in various conditions.
- Amiodarone does not need hospitalization for initiation.
- Long-term use of Amiodarone can cause pulmonary disease, hyperthyroidism, peripheral neuropathy etc.
- Long-term Amiodarone use may increase defibrillation threshold (energy needed for successful conversion of ventricular tachycardia).
- Sotalol reduces defibrillation threshold and thereby reducing the amount of energy needed for successful defibrillation.
- Because of the major renal excretory pathway, Sotalol is contraindicated for renal dysfunction.
- Calcium channel blockers are classified as class IV antiarrhythmics. They are divided into dihydropyridines (Nifedipine, Felodipine, Amlodipine) and non-dihydropyridines (Verapamil and Diltiazem).
- Non-dihydropyridine calcium channel blockers have electrophysiologic properties of prolonging AV node conduction and refractoriness.
- Calcium gluconate is the antidote for calcium channel blocker toxicity.
- Digoxin has a narrow therapeutic window of blood level (0.8 to 1.2 ng/ml).
- Digoxin should be avoided in patients with WPW pre-excitation because of the possible facilitation of impulse conduction through accessory pathway and resultant ventricular arrhythmia.
- Adenosine has no direct effect in the ventricle. Theophylline, which is an adenosine receptor blocking agents may prevent adenosine from working when used together.
- Adenosine has the potential for triggering atrial fibrillation.

Test Your Understanding

1. Which of the following represents a member of class III antiarrhythmics?
A   Flecainide
B   Carvedilol
C   Amiodarone
D   Procainamide

2. Which of the following best describes mechanism of action of Propafenone?
A   Potassium channel blocking
B   Calcium channel blocking
C   Beta blocking
D   Sodium channel blocking

3. Which of the following is the most potent sodium channel blocker?
A   Quinidine
B   Flecainide
C   Lidocaine
D   Mexiletine

4. Which of the following sodium channel blocking agents is useful in acute phase of ventricular arrhythmia secondary to myocardial infarction?
A   Procainamide
B   Amiodarone
C   Lidocaine
D   Flecainide

5. Which of the following is not an antiarrhythmic agent requiring in-hospital monitoring for initiation?
A   Sotalol
B   Procainamide
C   Amiodarone
D   Quinidine

6. Which of the following clinical condition is contraindicated for the use of Flecainide?
A   Non-critical atherosclerosis
B   Recent myocardial infarction
C   Peripheral vascular disease
D   Chronic hepatitis

7. Which of the following is an example for nonselective beta-blocker?
A   Carvedilol

B   Atenolol
C   Metoprolol
D   Esmolol

8. Which of the following statement is true regarding Sotalol?
A   It has only Class III properties
B   It increases defibrillation threshold
C   It has sodium and potassium blocking effect
D   Chronic use cause pulmonary fibrosis

9. Which of the following is an example for non-dihydropyridine calcium channel blocker?
A   Amlodipine
B   Nicardipine
C   Verapamil
D   Nifedipine

10. Digoxin is contraindicated in
_____?
A   Atrial fibrillation
B   Atrial flutter
C   Frequent PVCs
D   WPW syndrome

Answers

1.   C   Amiodarone
2.   D   Sodium channel blocking
3.   B   Flecainide
4.   C   Lidocaine
5.   C   Amiodarone
6.   B   Recent myocardial infarction
7.   A   Carvedilol
8.   C   It has sodium and potassium blocking effect
9.   C   Verapamil
10.   D   WPW syndrome

CHAPTER 15

Rhythm Practice

In this chapter

- Single rhythm practice
- 12 lead EKG practice

Most of these rhythm strips and EKG tracings are taken from real patients in various cardiac monitoring settings. Therefore, some of the strips have motion artifact along with underlying rhythm, which can be a bit confusing unless the interpreter is careful. We have done it on purpose to provide a realistic view of EKG interpretation in the field.

Individual Rhythm Strips

1.

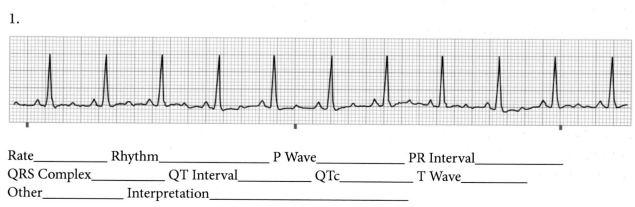

Rate_____ Rhythm_____ P Wave_____ PR Interval_____
QRS Complex_____ QT Interval_____ QTc_____ T Wave_____
Other_____ Interpretation_____

2.

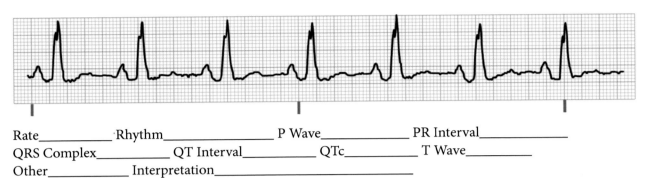

Rate_____ Rhythm_____ P Wave_____ PR Interval_____
QRS Complex_____ QT Interval_____ QTc_____ T Wave_____
Other_____ Interpretation_____

3.

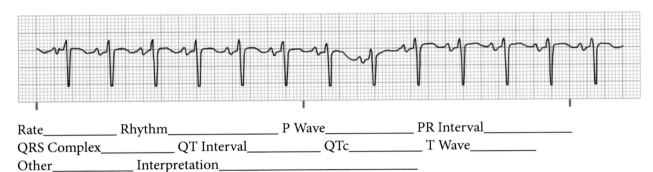

Rate_____ Rhythm_____ P Wave_____ PR Interval_____
QRS Complex_____ QT Interval_____ QTc_____ T Wave_____
Other_____ Interpretation_____

4.

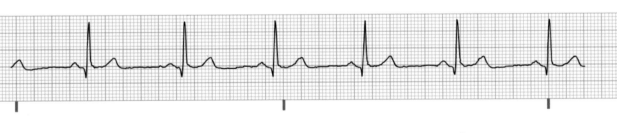

Rate_____ Rhythm_____ P Wave_____ PR Interval_____
QRS Complex_____ QT Interval_____ QTc_____ T Wave_____
Other_____ Interpretation_____

5.

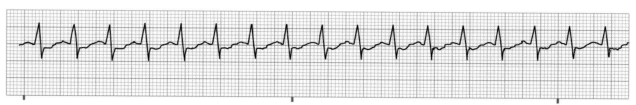

Rate_____ Rhythm_____ P Wave_____ PR Interval_____
QRS Complex_____ QT Interval_____ QTc_____ T Wave_____
Other_____ Interpretation_____

6.

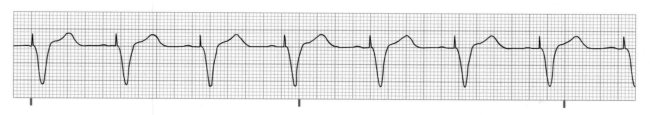

Rate_____ Rhythm_____ P Wave_____ PR Interval_____
QRS Complex_____ QT Interval_____ QTc_____ T Wave_____
Other_____ Interpretation_____

7.

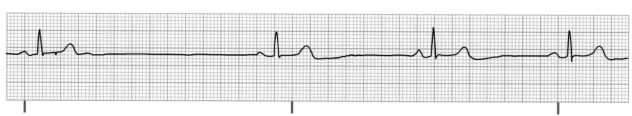

Rate_____ Rhythm_____ P Wave_____ PR Interval_____
QRS Complex_____ QT Interval_____ QTc_____ T Wave_____
Other_____ Interpretation_____

8.

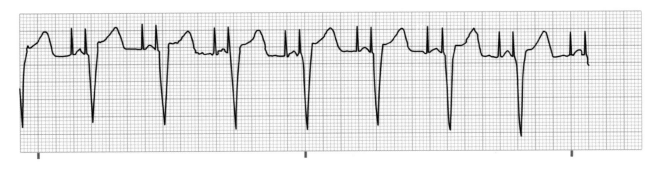

Rate_____ Rhythm_____ P Wave_____ PR Interval_____
QRS Complex_____ QT Interval_____ QTc_____ T Wave_____
Other_____ Interpretation_____

9.

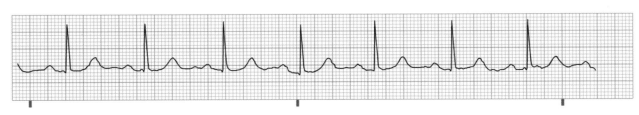

Rate_____ Rhythm_____ P Wave_____ PR Interval_____
QRS Complex_____ QT Interval_____ QTc_____ T Wave_____
Other_____ Interpretation_____

10.

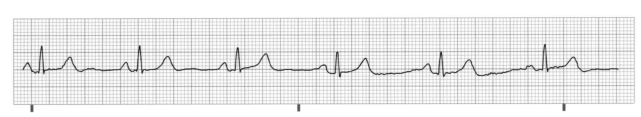

Rate_____ Rhythm_____ P Wave_____ PR Interval_____
QRS Complex_____ QT Interval_____ QTc_____ T Wave_____
Other_____ Interpretation_____

11.

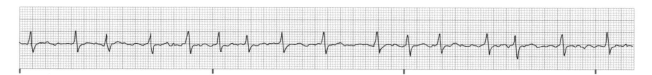

Rate_____ Rhythm_____ P Wave_____ PR Interval_____
QRS Complex_____ QT Interval_____ QTc_____ T Wave_____
Other_____ Interpretation_____

12.

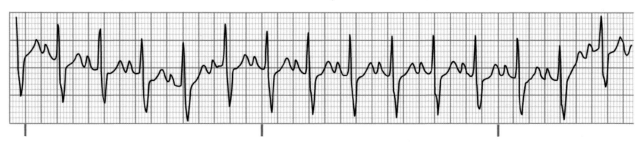

Rate_____ Rhythm_____ P Wave_____ PR Interval_____
QRS Complex_____ QT Interval_____ QTc_____ T Wave_____
Other_____ Interpretation_____

13.

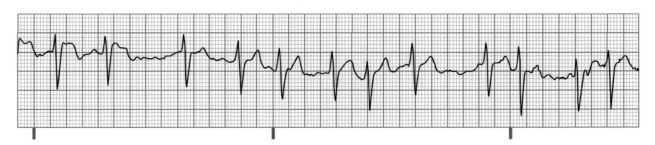

Rate_____ Rhythm_____ P Wave_____ PR Interval_____
QRS Complex_____ QT Interval_____ QTc_____ T Wave_____
Other_____ Interpretation_____

14.

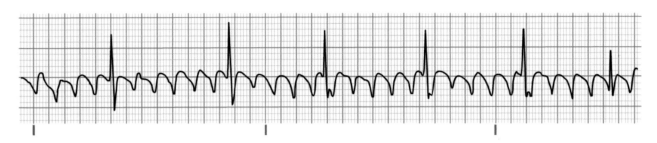

Rate_____ Rhythm_____ P Wave_____ PR Interval_____
QRS Complex_____ QT Interval_____ QTc_____ T Wave_____
Other_____ Interpretation_____

15.

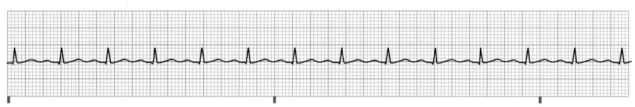

Rate_____ Rhythm_____ P Wave_____ PR Interval_____
QRS Complex_____ QT Interval_____ QTc_____ T Wave_____
Other_____ Interpretation_____

16.

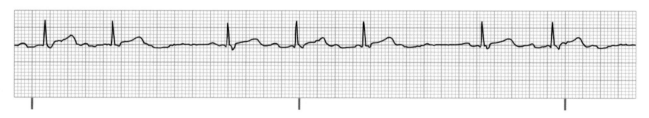

Rate_____ Rhythm_____ P Wave_____ PR Interval_____
QRS Complex_____ QT Interval_____ QTc_____ T Wave_____
Other_____ Interpretation_____

17.

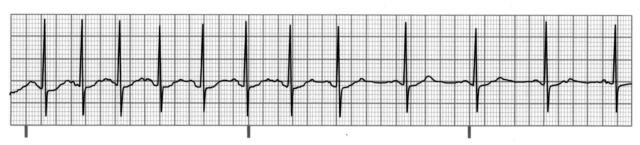

Rate_____ Rhythm_____ P Wave_____ PR Interval_____
QRS Complex_____ QT Interval_____ QTc_____ T Wave_____
Other_____ Interpretation_____

18.

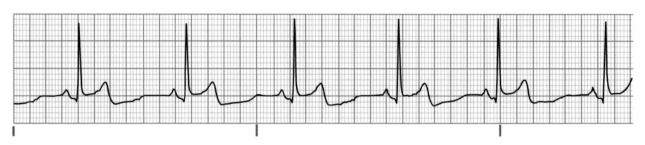

Rate_____ Rhythm_____ P Wave_____ PR Interval_____
QRS Complex_____ QT Interval_____ QTc_____ T Wave_____
Other_____ Interpretation_____

19.

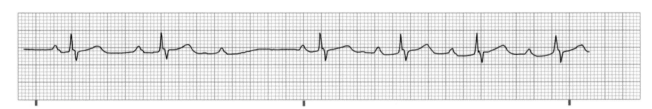

Rate_____ Rhythm_____ P Wave_____ PR Interval_____
QRS Complex_____ QT Interval_____ QTc_____ T Wave_____
Other_____ Interpretation_____

20.

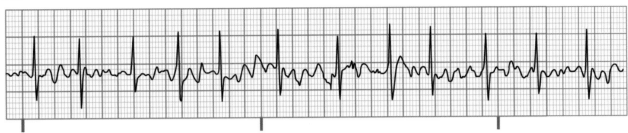

Rate_____ Rhythm_____ P Wave_____ PR Interval_____
QRS Complex_____ QT Interval_____ QTc_____ T Wave_____
Other_____ Interpretation_____

21.

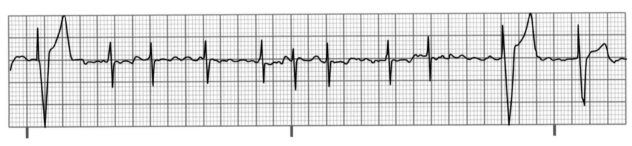

Rate_____ Rhythm_____ P Wave_____ PR Interval_____
QRS Complex_____ QT Interval_____ QTc_____ T Wave_____
Other_____ Interpretation_____

22.

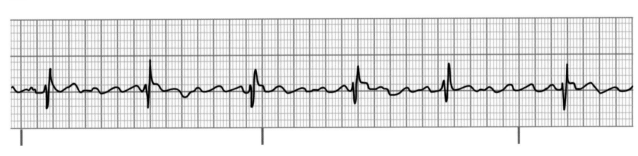

Rate_____ Rhythm_____ P Wave_____ PR Interval_____
QRS Complex_____ QT Interval_____ QTc_____ T Wave_____
Other_____ Interpretation_____

23.

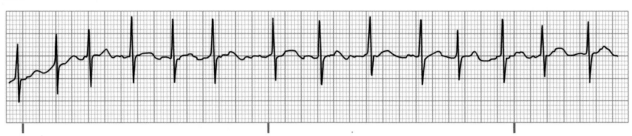

Rate_____ Rhythm_____ P Wave_____ PR Interval_____

QRS Complex_____ QT Interval_____ QTc_____ T Wave_____

Other_____ Interpretation_____

24.

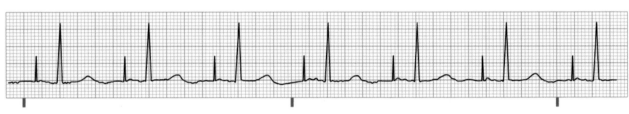

Rate_____ Rhythm_____ P Wave_____ PR Interval_____

QRS Complex_____ QT Interval_____ QTc_____ T Wave_____

Other_____ Interpretation_____

25.

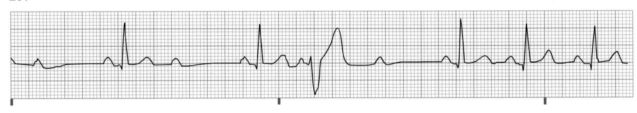

Rate_____ Rhythm_____ P Wave_____ PR Interval_____

QRS Complex_____ QT Interval_____ QTc_____ T Wave_____

Other_____ Interpretation_____

26.

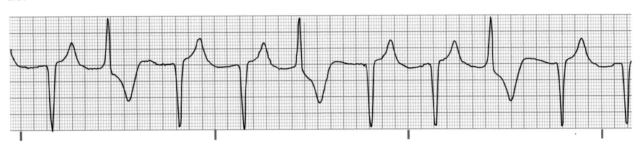

Rate_____ Rhythm_____ P Wave_____ PR Interval_____
QRS Complex_____ QT Interval_____ QTc_____ T Wave_____
Other_____ Interpretation_____

27.

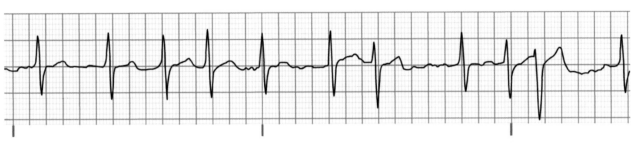

Rate_____ Rhythm_____ P Wave_____ PR Interval_____
QRS Complex_____ QT Interval_____ QTc_____ T Wave_____
Other_____ Interpretation_____

28.

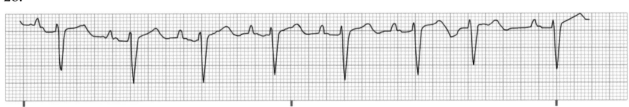

Rate_____ Rhythm_____ P Wave_____ PR Interval_____
QRS Complex_____ QT Interval_____ QTc_____ T Wave_____
Other_____ Interpretation_____

29.

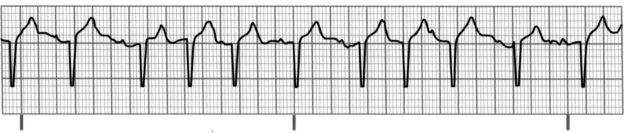

Rate_____ Rhythm_____ P Wave_____ PR Interval_____
QRS Complex_____ QT Interval_____ QTc_____ T Wave_____
Other_____ Interpretation_____

30.

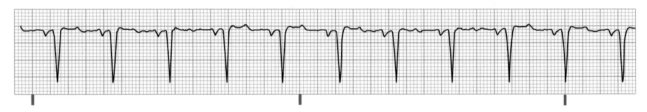

Rate_____ Rhythm_____ P Wave_____ PR Interval_____
QRS Complex_____ QT Interval_____ QTc_____ T Wave_____
Other_____ Interpretation_____

31.

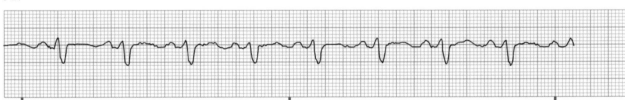

Rate_____ Rhythm_____ P Wave_____ PR Interval_____
QRS Complex_____ QT Interval_____ QTc_____ T Wave_____
Other_____ Interpretation_____

32.

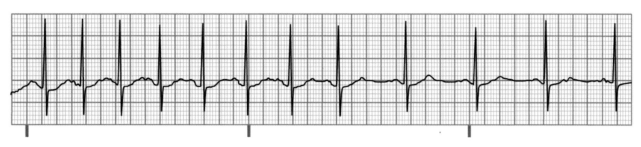

Rate_____ Rhythm_____ P Wave_____ PR Interval_____

QRS Complex_____ QT Interval_____ QTc_____ T Wave_____

Other_____ Interpretation_____

33.

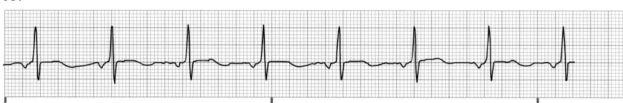

Rate_____ Rhythm_____ P Wave_____ PR Interval_____

QRS Complex_____ QT Interval_____ QTc_____ T Wave_____

Other_____ Interpretation_____

34.

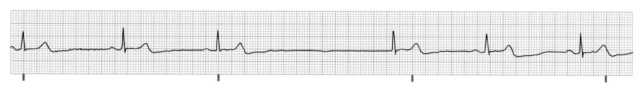

Rate_____ Rhythm_____ P Wave_____ PR Interval_____

QRS Complex_____ QT Interval_____ QTc_____ T Wave_____

Other_____ Interpretation_____

35.

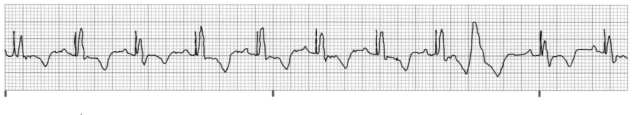

Rate_____ Rhythm_____ P Wave_____ PR Interval_____
QRS Complex_____ QT Interval_____ QTc_____ T Wave_____
Other_____ Interpretation_____

36.

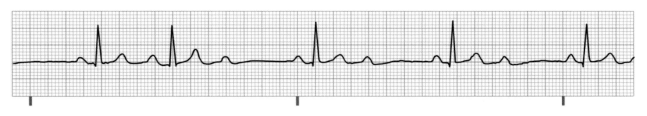

Rate_____ Rhythm_____ P Wave_____ PR Interval_____
QRS Complex_____ QT Interval_____ QTc_____ T Wave_____
Other_____ Interpretation_____

37.

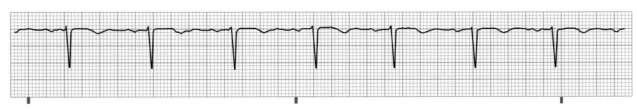

Rate_____ Rhythm_____ P Wave_____ PR Interval_____
QRS Complex_____ QT Interval_____ QTc_____ T Wave_____
Other_____ Interpretation_____

38.

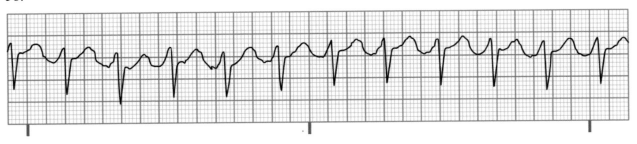

Rate_____ Rhythm_____ P Wave_____ PR Interval_____
QRS Complex_____ QT Interval_____ QTc_____ T Wave_____
Other_____ Interpretation_____

39.

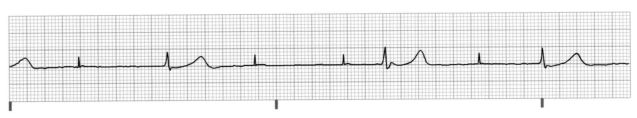

Rate_____ Rhythm_____ P Wave_____ PR Interval_____
QRS Complex_____ QT Interval_____ QTc_____ T Wave_____
Other_____ Interpretation_____

40.

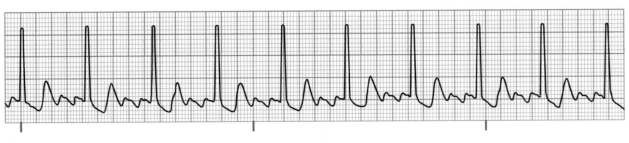

Rate_____ Rhythm_____ P Wave_____ PR Interval_____
QRS Complex_____ QT Interval_____ QTc_____ T Wave_____
Other_____ Interpretation_____

41.

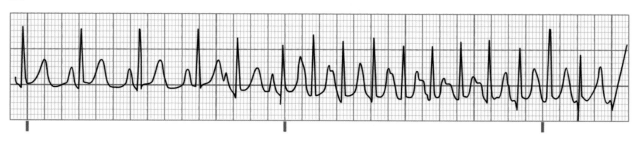

Rate_____ Rhythm_____ P Wave_____ PR Interval_____
QRS Complex_____ QT Interval_____ QTc_____ T Wave_____
Other_____ Interpretation_____

42.

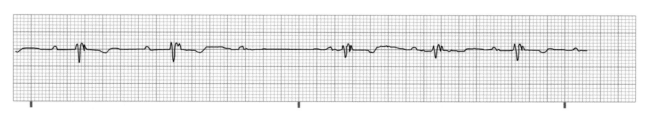

Rate_____ Rhythm_____ P Wave_____ PR Interval_____
QRS Complex_____ QT Interval_____ QTc_____ T Wave_____
Other_____ Interpretation_____

43.

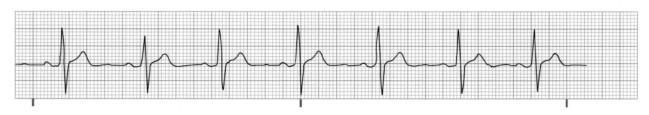

Rate_____ Rhythm_____ P Wave_____ PR Interval_____
QRS Complex_____ QT Interval_____ QTc_____ T Wave_____
Other_____ Interpretation_____

44.

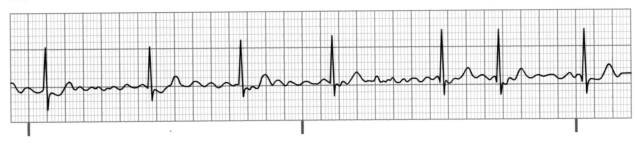

Rate_____ Rhythm_____ P Wave_____ PR Interval_____
QRS Complex_____ QT Interval_____ QTc_____ T Wave_____
Other_____ Interpretation_____

45.

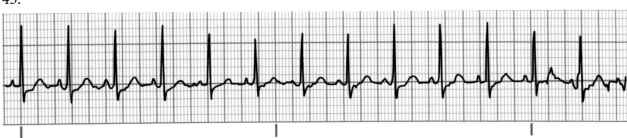

Rate_____ Rhythm_____ P Wave_____ PR Interval_____
QRS Complex_____ QT Interval_____ QTc_____ T Wave_____
Other_____ Interpretation_____

46.

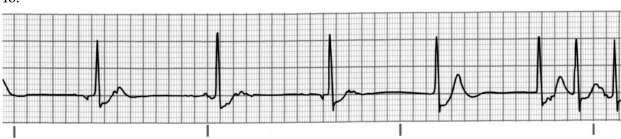

Rate_____ Rhythm_____ P Wave_____ PR Interval_____
QRS Complex_____ QT Interval_____ QTc_____ T Wave_____
Other_____ Interpretation_____

47.

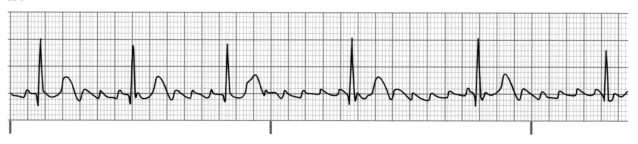

Rate_____ Rhythm_____ P Wave_____ PR Interval_____
QRS Complex_____ QT Interval_____ QTc_____ T Wave_____
Other_____ Interpretation_____

48.

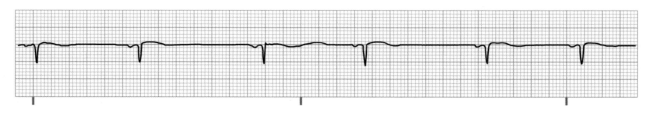

Rate_____ Rhythm_____ P Wave_____ PR Interval_____
QRS Complex_____ QT Interval_____ QTc_____ T Wave_____
Other_____ Interpretation_____

49.

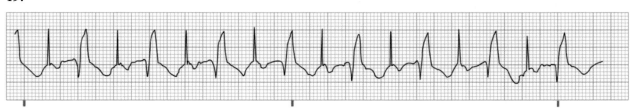

Rate_____ Rhythm_____ P Wave_____ PR Interval_____
QRS Complex_____ QT Interval_____ QTc_____ T Wave_____
Other_____ Interpretation_____

50.

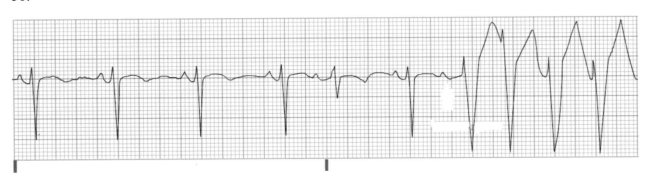

Rate_____ Rhythm_____ P Wave_____ PR Interval_____

QRS Complex_____ QT Interval_____ QTc_____ T Wave_____

Other_____ Interpretation_____

51.

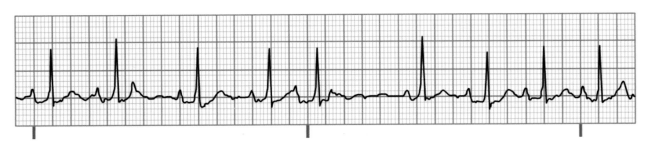

Rate_____ Rhythm_____ P Wave_____ PR Interval_____

QRS Complex_____ QT Interval_____ QTc_____ T Wave_____

Other_____ Interpretation_____

52.

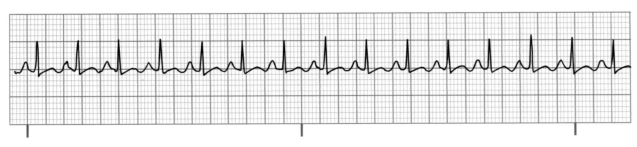

Rate_____ Rhythm_____ P Wave_____ PR Interval_____

QRS Complex_____ QT Interval_____ QTc_____ T Wave_____

Other_____ Interpretation_____

53.

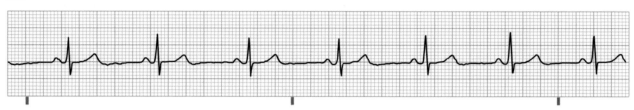

Rate_____ Rhythm_____ P Wave_____ PR Interval_____

QRS Complex_____ QT Interval_____ QTc_____ T Wave_____

Other_____ Interpretation_____

54.

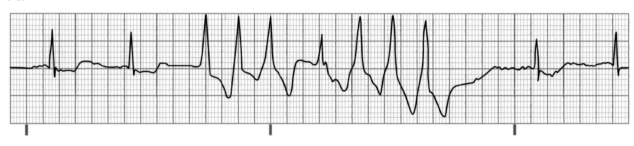

Rate_____ Rhythm_____ P Wave_____ PR Interval_____

QRS Complex_____ QT Interval_____ QTc_____ T Wave_____

Other_____ Interpretation_____

55.

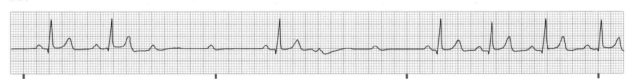

Rate_____ Rhythm_____ P Wave_____ PR Interval_____

QRS Complex_____ QT Interval_____ QTc_____ T Wave_____

Other_____ Interpretation_____

56.

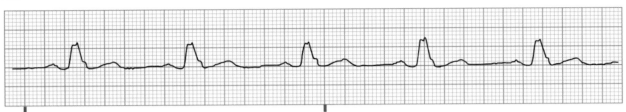

Rate_____ Rhythm_____ P Wave_____ PR Interval_____
QRS Complex_____ QT Interval_____ QTc_____ T Wave_____
Other_____ Interpretation_____

57.

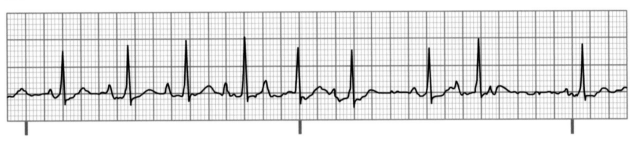

Rate_____ Rhythm_____ P Wave_____ PR Interval_____
QRS Complex_____ QT Interval_____ QTc_____ T Wave_____
Other_____ Interpretation_____

58.

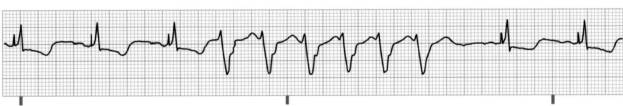

Rate_____ Rhythm_____ P Wave_____ PR Interval_____
QRS Complex_____ QT Interval_____ QTc_____ T Wave_____
Other_____ Interpretation_____

59.

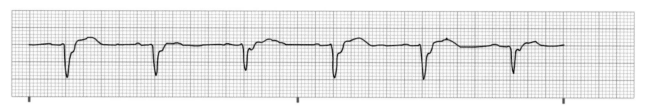

Rate_____ Rhythm_____ P Wave_____ PR Interval_____

QRS Complex_____ QT Interval_____ QTc_____ T Wave_____

Other_____ Interpretation_____

60.

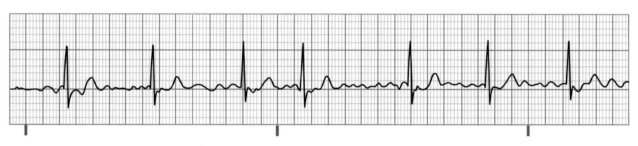

Rate_____ Rhythm_____ P Wave_____ PR Interval_____

QRS Complex_____ QT Interval_____ QTc_____ T Wave_____

Other_____ Interpretation_____

12 Lead EKG Practice

1.

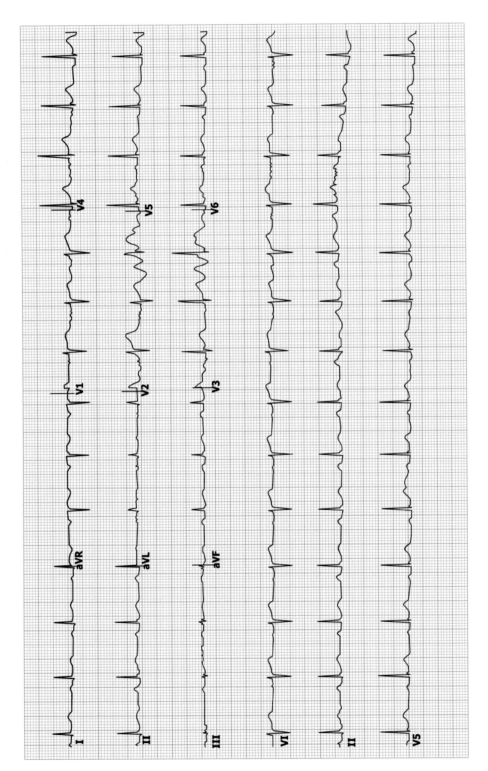

Rate Rhythm		Enlargement of Atria/ Ventricle	
Axis		Ischemia/ Infarction	
Bundle block/ Hemiblock		Other abnormalities	
Interpretation			

2.

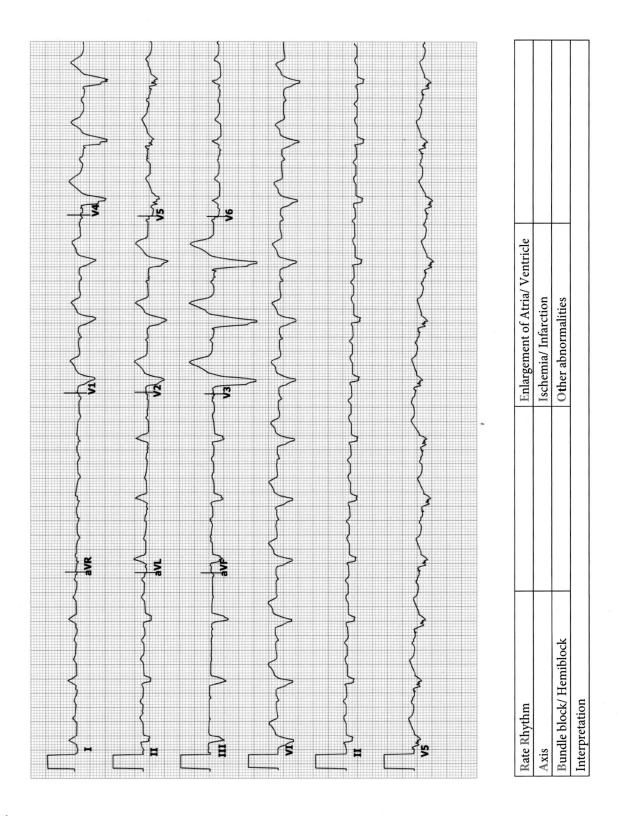

Rate Rhythm		Enlargement of Atria/ Ventricle	
Axis		Ischemia/ Infarction	
Bundle block/ Hemiblock		Other abnormalities	
Interpretation			

3.

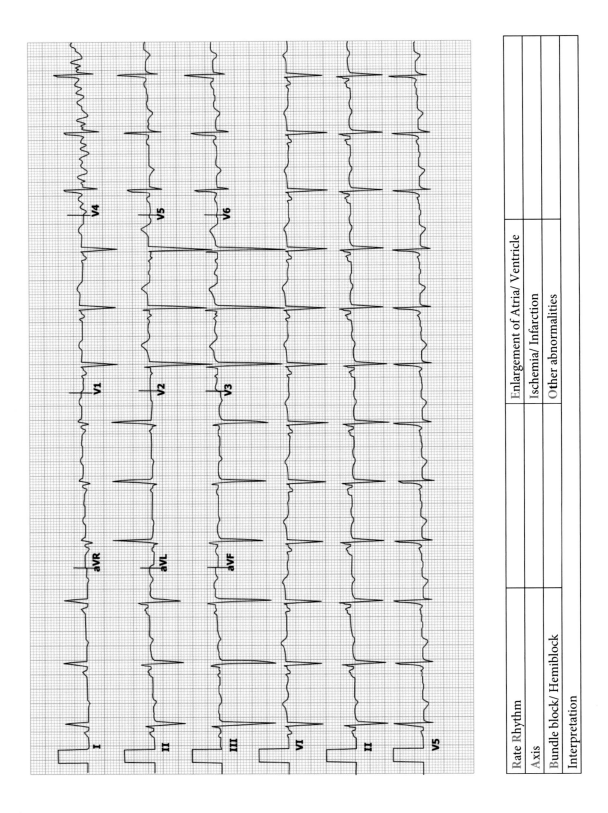

Rate Rhythm		Enlargement of Atria/ Ventricle	
Axis		Ischemia/ Infarction	
Bundle block/ Hemiblock		Other abnormalities	
Interpretation			

4.

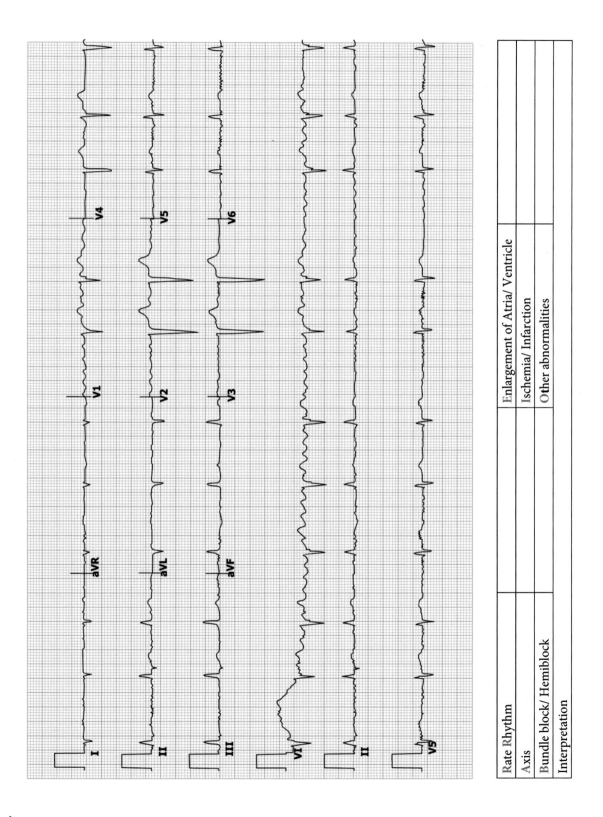

Rate Rhythm		Enlargement of Atria/ Ventricle	
Axis		Ischemia/ Infarction	
Bundle block/ Hemiblock		Other abnormalities	
Interpretation			

5.

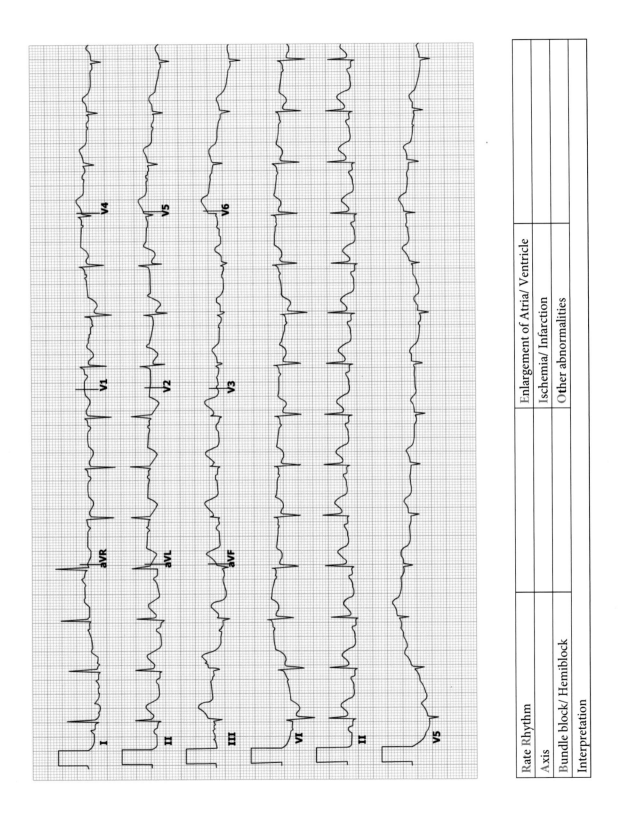

Rate Rhythm		Enlargement of Atria/ Ventricle	
Axis		Ischemia/ Infarction	
Bundle block/ Hemiblock		Other abnormalities	
Interpretation			

6.

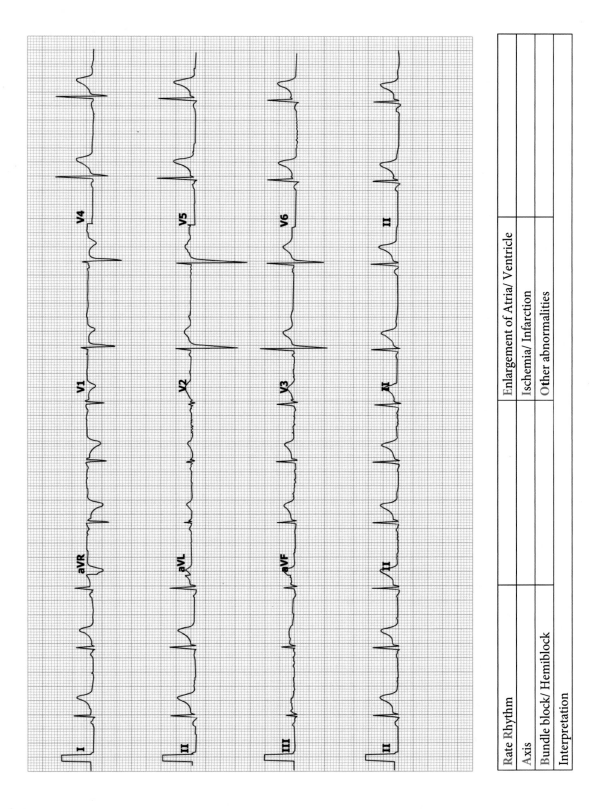

Rate Rhythm		Enlargement of Atria/ Ventricle	
Axis		Ischemia/ Infarction	
Bundle block/ Hemiblock		Other abnormalities	
Interpretation			

7.

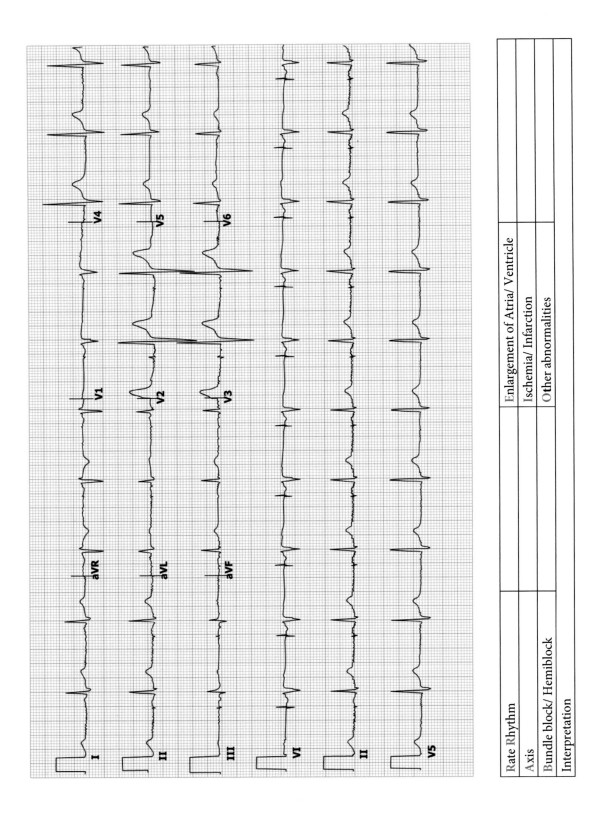

Rate Rhythm		Enlargement of Atria/ Ventricle	
Axis		Ischemia/ Infarction	
Bundle block/ Hemiblock		Other abnormalities	
Interpretation			

8.

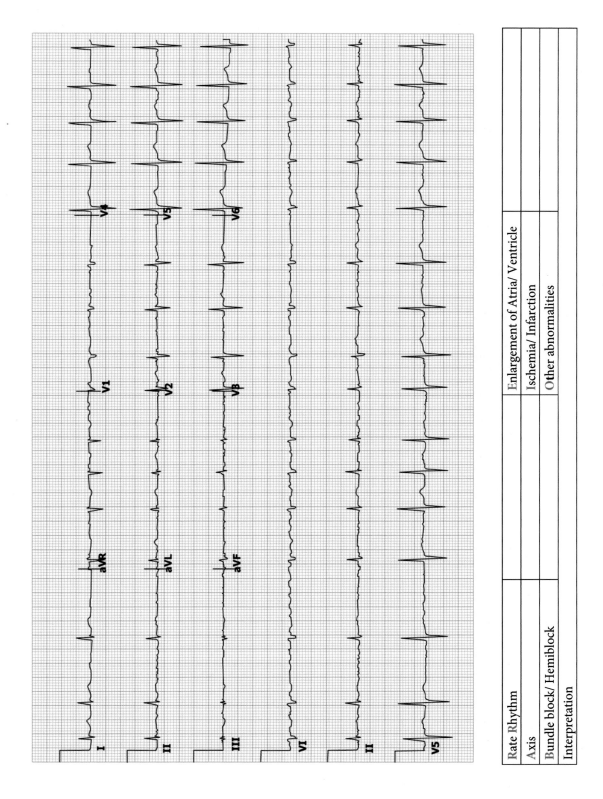

Rate Rhythm		Enlargement of Atria/ Ventricle	
Axis		Ischemia/ Infarction	
Bundle block/ Hemiblock		Other abnormalities	
Interpretation			

9.

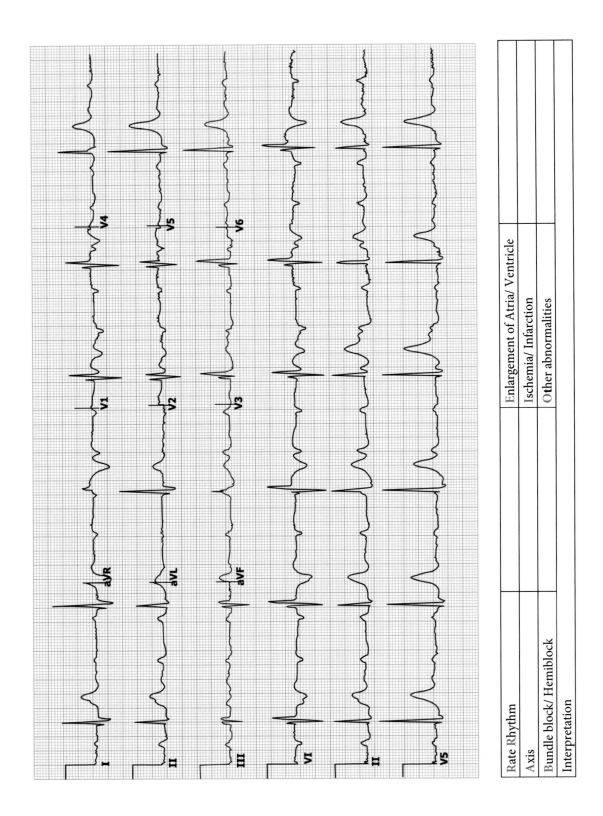

Rate Rhythm			Enlargement of Atria/ Ventricle	
Axis			Ischemia/ Infarction	
Bundle block/ Hemiblock			Other abnormalities	
Interpretation				

10.

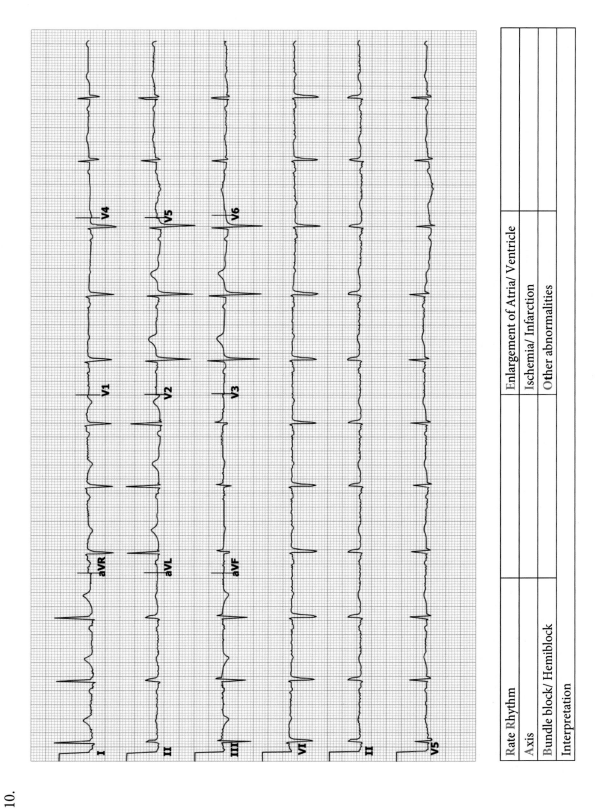

	Enlargement of Atria/ Ventricle		
Rate Rhythm			
Axis	Ischemia/ Infarction		
Bundle block/ Hemiblock	Other abnormalities		
Interpretation			

11.

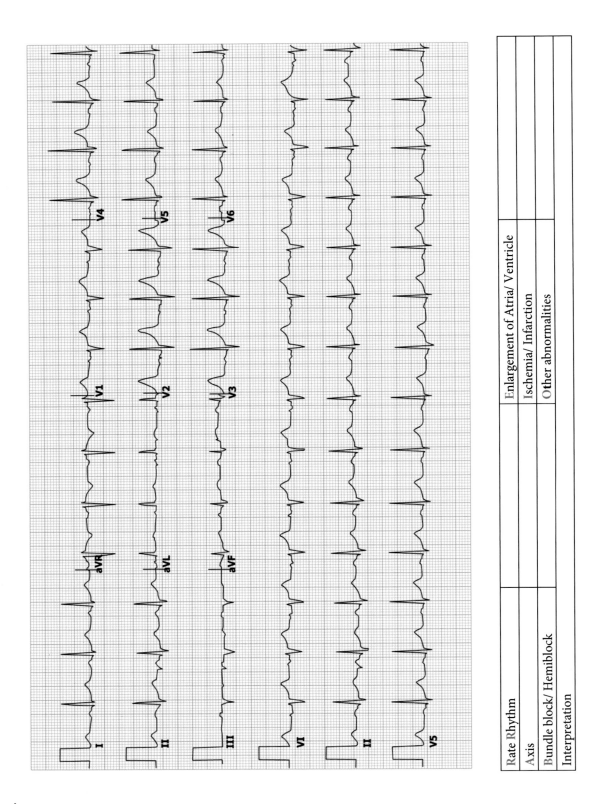

Rate Rhythm		Enlargement of Atria/ Ventricle	
Axis		Ischemia/ Infarction	
Bundle block/ Hemiblock		Other abnormalities	
Interpretation			

12.

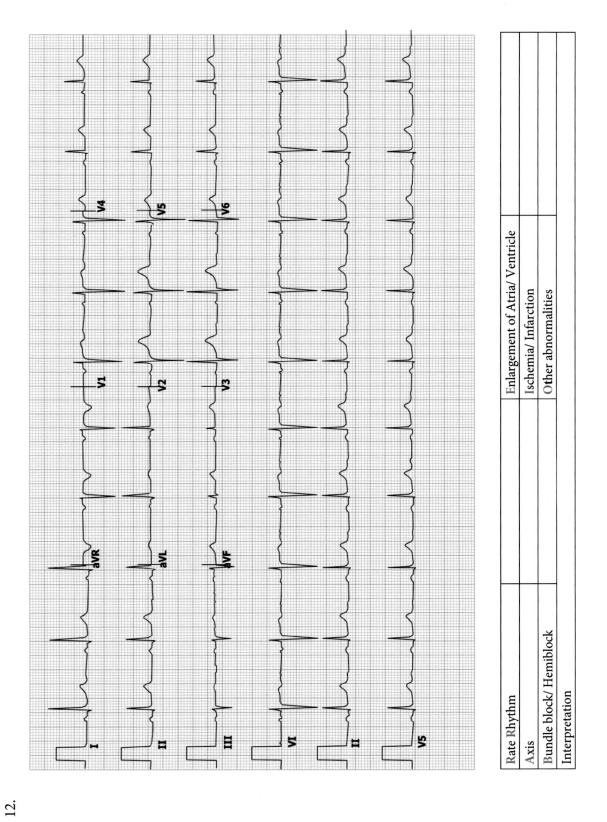

Rate Rhythm		Enlargement of Atria/ Ventricle	
Axis		Ischemia/ Infarction	
Bundle block/ Hemiblock		Other abnormalities	
Interpretation			

13.

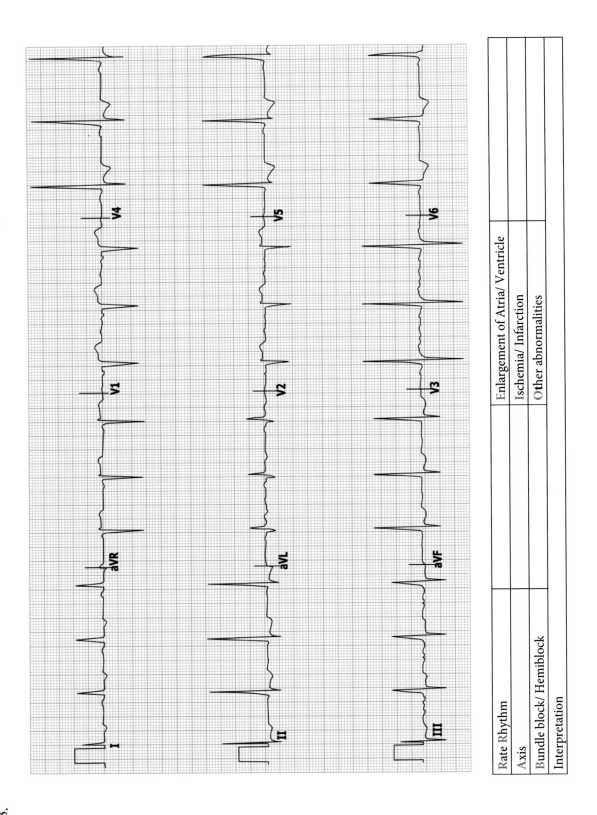

Rate Rhythm			
Axis			
Bundle block/ Hemiblock			
Interpretation			

	Enlargement of Atria/ Ventricle	
	Ischemia/ Infarction	
	Other abnormalities	

14.

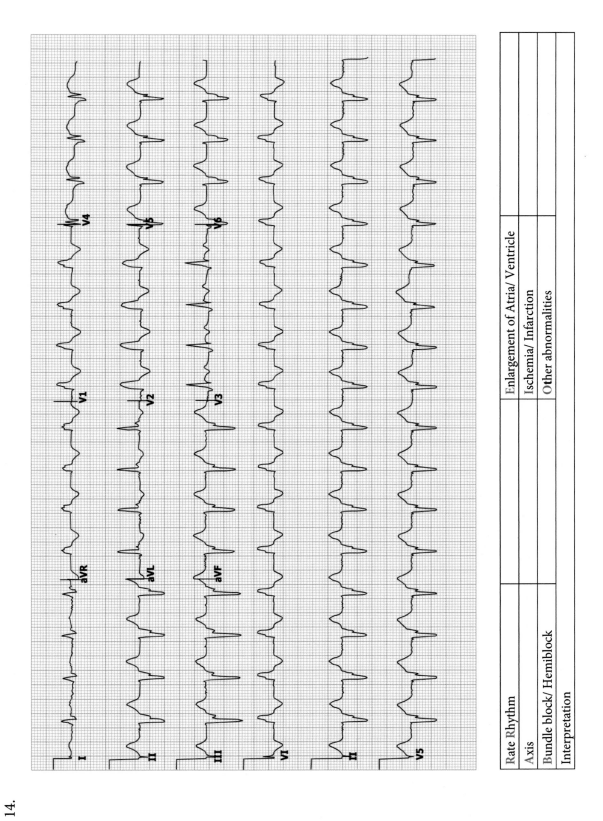

Rate Rhythm		Enlargement of Atria/ Ventricle	
Axis		Ischemia/ Infarction	
Bundle block/ Hemiblock		Other abnormalities	
Interpretation			

15.

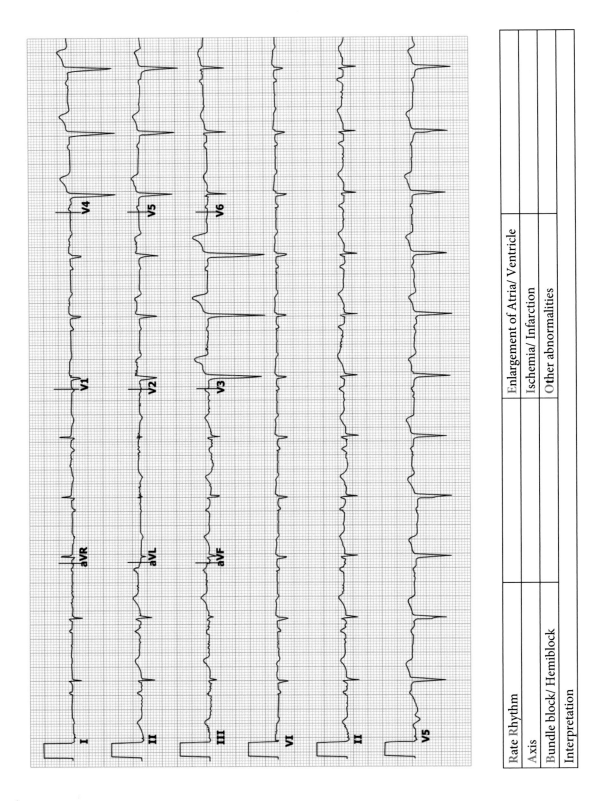

Rate Rhythm		Enlargement of Atria/ Ventricle	
Axis		Ischemia/ Infarction	
Bundle block/ Hemiblock		Other abnormalities	
Interpretation			

16.

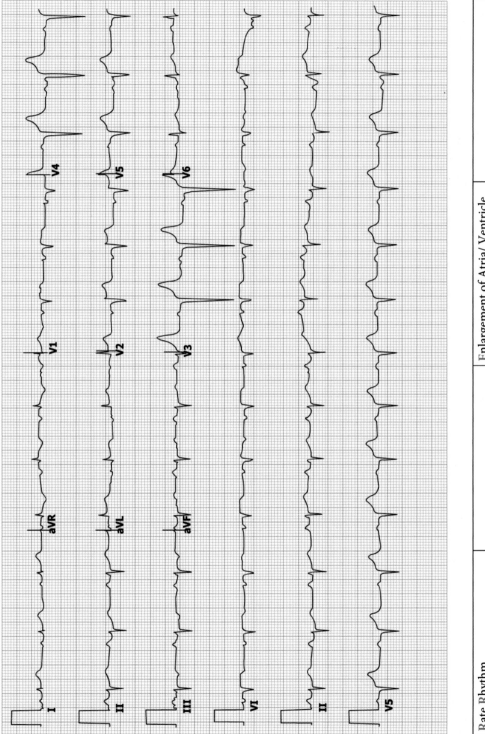

Rate Rhythm		Enlargement of Atria/ Ventricle	
Axis		Ischemia/ Infarction	
Bundle block/ Hemiblock		Other abnormalities	
Interpretation			

17.

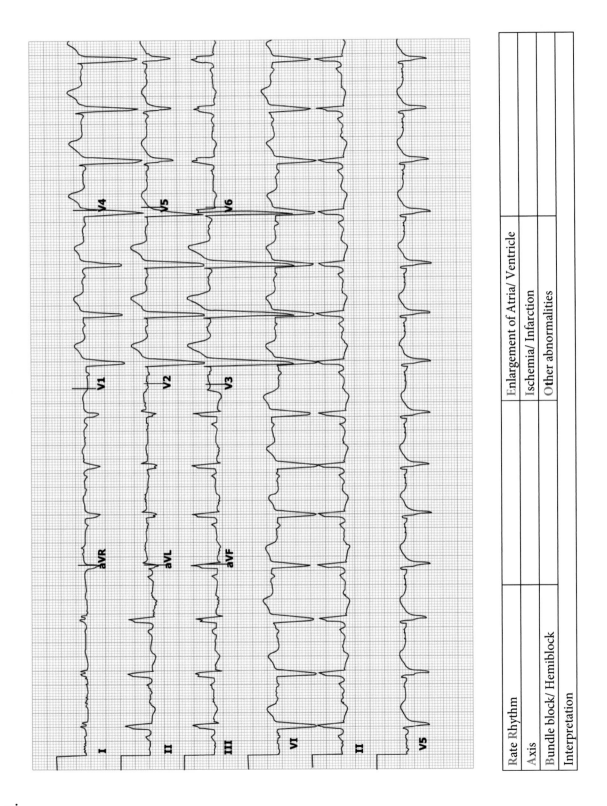

Rate Rhythm		Enlargement of Atria/ Ventricle	
Axis		Ischemia/ Infarction	
Bundle block/ Hemiblock		Other abnormalities	
Interpretation			

18.

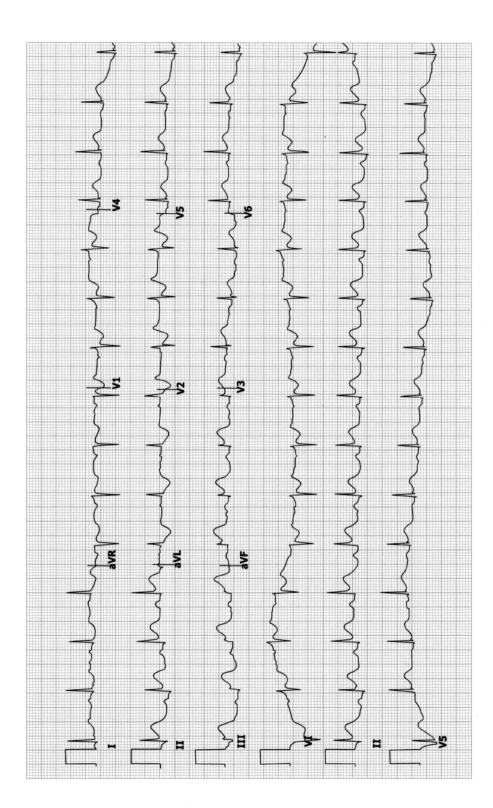

Rate Rhythm		Enlargement of Atria/ Ventricle	
Axis		Ischemia/ Infarction	
Bundle block/ Hemiblock		Other abnormalities	
Interpretation			

19.

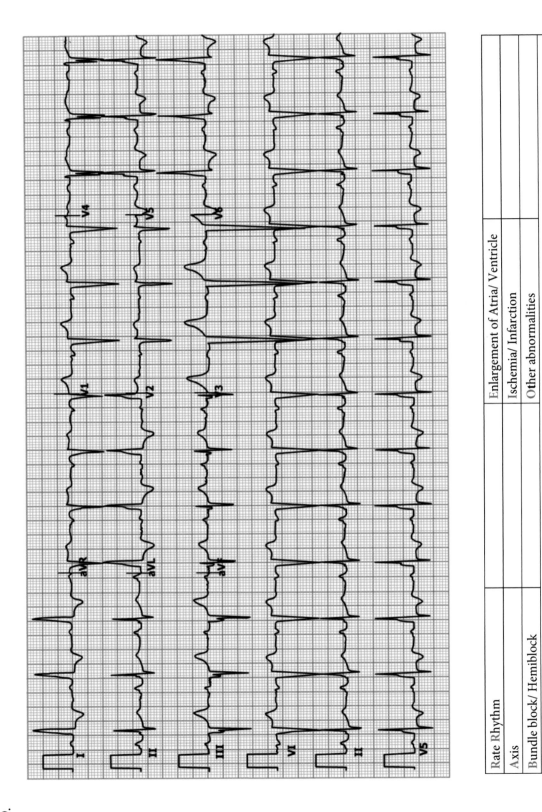

Rate Rhythm		Enlargement of Atria/ Ventricle	
Axis		Ischemia/ Infarction	
Bundle block/ Hemiblock		Other abnormalities	
Interpretation			

20.

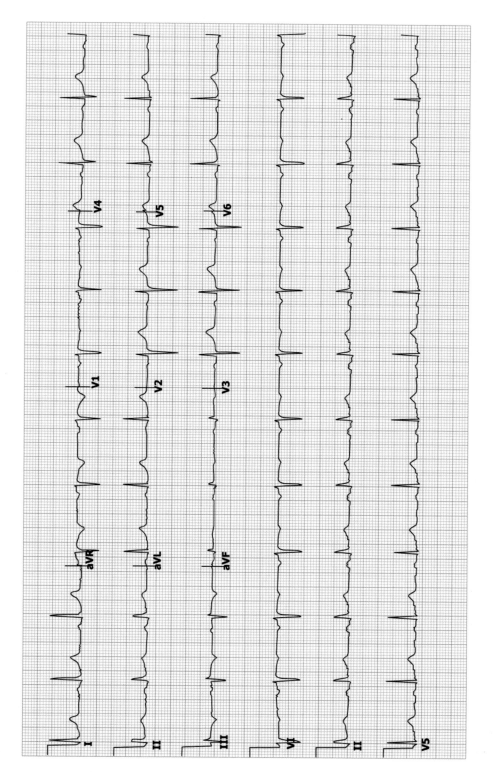

Rate Rhythm		Enlargement of Atria/ Ventricle	
Axis		Ischemia/ Infarction	
Bundle block/ Hemiblock		Other abnormalities	
Interpretation			

Answer Key

Individual lead interpretation

1. Rate __93 BPM ___ Rhythm __regular rhythm ___ P Wave _present ___PR Interval __0.14 seconds ___ QRS Complex _narrow __ QT Interval__0.34 seconds ___ QTc__0.439 seconds ___ T Wave _present _ Other __none __ Interpretation __normal sinus rhythm _____

2. Rate __63 BPM ___ Rhythm __regular rhythm ___ P Wave _present ___PR Interval __0.22 seconds ___ QRS Complex _wide- 0.14 second__ QT Interval__0.48 seconds___ QTc__0.49 seconds___ T Wave _present _ Other __possible bundle branch__ Interpretation __normal sinus rhythm with bundle branch block _____

3. Rate __125 BPM ___ Rhythm __regular rhythm ___ P Wave _present ___PR Interval __0. 16 seconds ___ QRS Complex _narrow __ QT Interval__0. 26 seconds ___ QTc__0.368 seconds ___ T Wave _present _ Other __tachycardia__ Interpretation __sinus tachycardia_____

4. Rate __58 BPM ___ Rhythm __regular rhythm ___ P Wave _present ___PR Interval __0. 20 seconds ___ QRS Complex _narrow __ QT Interval__0. 42 seconds ___ QTc__0.412 seconds ___ T Wave _present _ Other __presence of Q wave__ Interpretation __sinus bradycardia with prominent Q wave_____

5. Rate __166 BPM ___ Rhythm __regular___ P Wave _present but sometimes buried ___PR Interval __ 0.14 when present___ QRS Complex _narrow __ QT Interval__0.22 seconds ___ QTc __0.367 seconds ___ T Wave _present but distorted with P wave _ Other __tachycardia __ Interpretation __supraventricular tachycardia _____

6. . Rate __65 BPM ___ Rhythm __regular ___ P Wave _present ___PR Interval __0.20 seconds ___ QRS Complex _0.16 seconds __ QT Interval__0.52 seconds ___ QTc __0.536 seconds ___ T Wave _present _ Other __pacer spikes __ Interpretation __ventricular paced rhythm _____

7. . Rate __30's ___ Rhythm __irregular ___ P Wave _present ___PR Interval __0.20 seconds ___ QRS Complex _0.06 seconds__ QT Interval__0.42 seconds ___ QTc __not measured___ T Wave _present _ Other __present of 2.68 seconds pause __ Interpretation __sinus bradycardia with 2.68 second pause_____

8. . Rate __75 BPM ___ Rhythm __regular___ P Wave _present ___PR Interval __0.18 seconds ___ QRS Complex _0.1 server seconds __ QT Interval__0.42 seconds___ QTc __0.424 seconds___ T Wave _present _ Other __presence of pacer spikes __ Interpretation __AV paced rhythm _____

9. . Rate __68 BPM ___ Rhythm __regular___ P Wave _present ___PR Interval __0.24 seconds ___ QRS Complex _narrow __ QT Interval__0.44 seconds ___ QTc __0.469 seconds ___ T Wave _present _ Other __long PR interval __ Interpretation __sinus rhythm with a first degree heart block _____

10. . Rate __55 BPM ___ Rhythm __regular ___ P Wave _present ___PR Interval __0.20 seconds ___QRS Complex _narrow __ QT Interval__0.44 seconds ___ QTc __0.416 seconds ___ T Wave _present _ Other __none __ Interpretation __sinus bradycardia _____

11. . Rate __100's BPM ___ Rhythm __irregular___ P Wave _multiple undulating P waves ___PR Interval __not measurable ___ QRS Complex _narrow __ QT Interval__ not measurable ___ QTc __not measurable___ T Wave _ present but distorted with P waves_ Other __none __ Interpretation __atrial fibrillation with rapid ventricular response_____

12. Rate __115 BPM ___ Rhythm __regular ___ P Wave _present ___PR Interval __0.18 seconds ___ QRS Complex _0.12seconds __ QT Interval__0.38 seconds ___ QTc __0.527seconds ___ T Wave _present _ Other __ __ Interpretation __sinus tachycardia with possible bundle branch block _____

13. . Rate __90's BPM ___ Rhythm __irregular___ P Wave _multiple and undulating ___PR Interval __not measurable ___ QRS Complex _0.12 seconds __ QT Interval__0.36 seconds ___ QTc __0.398 seconds ___ T Wave _present but distorted with P waves_ Other __none __ Interpretation __atrial fibrillation with controlled ventricular response and possible bundle branch block _____

14. . Rate __40's BPM ___ Rhythm __irregular___ P Wave _multiple saw tooth shaped P waves ___PR Interval __not measurable___ QRS Complex _narrow__ QT Interval__ unable to calculate___ QTc __not measurable___ T Wave _present but deformed by P waves_ Other __none __ Interpretation __atrial flutter with variable conduction block _____

15. . Rate __115 BPM ___ Rhythm __regular ___ P Wave _present ___PR Interval __0.20 seconds ___ QRS Complex _narrow __ QT Interval__0.28 seconds ___ QTc __0.388 seconds ___ T Wave _present _ Other __none __ Interpretation __sinus tachycardia _____

16. . Rate __70's BPM ___ Rhythm __irregular ___ P Wave _present ___PR Interval __variable ___ QRS Complex _ narrow__ QT Interval__0.38 seconds ___ QTc __not measured___ T Wave _absent in missing waves _ Other __missing QRS complex __ Interpretation __sinus rhythm with second-degree type I (Mobitz type I) heart block_____

17. . Rate __115 BPM in tachycardia and 65BPM in regular rhythm ___ Rhythm __regular with tachycardia ___ P Wave _present but not always seen in tachycardia ___PR Interval __0.20 seconds ___ QRS Complex _narrow __ QT Interval__ 0.44 seconds in regular rhythm and not measurable during tachycardia ___ QTc __0.464 seconds in regular rhythm___ T Wave _present _ Other __tachycardia turns to regular rhythm __ Interpretation __paroxysmal supraventricular tachycardia changing to sinus rhythm_____

18. . Rate __45 BPM ___ Rhythm __regular ___ P Wave _present ___PR Interval __0.20 seconds ___ QRS Complex _narrow __ QT Interval__0.44 seconds ___ QTc __0.377 seconds ___ T Wave _present _ Other __none __ Interpretation __sinus bradycardia _____

19. . Rate __60's BPM ___ Rhythm __irregular ___ P Wave _present ___PR Interval __variable ___ QRS Complex _missing in between__ QT Interval__.44 seconds___ QTc __not measured___ T Wave _missing in between _ Other __progressive drop in QRS __ Interpretation __sinus rhythm with second-degree type I (Mobitz type I) heart block _____

20. . Rate __ 100's BPM ___ Rhythm __ irregular___ P Wave _multiple and undulating ___PR Interval __not measurable ___ QRS Complex _narrow __ QT Interval__ not measurable___ QTc __not measurable___ T Wave _ distorted by P wave_ Other __none__ Interpretation __atrial fibrillation with rapid ventricular response _____

21. . Rate __100's BPM ___ Rhythm __irregular ___ P Wave _multiple and undulating ___PR Interval __not measurable ___ QRS Complex _narrow except during PVC __ QT Interval __not measurable___ QTc __not measurable___ T Wave _present but distorted by P wave _ Other __ none __ Interpretation __atrial fibrillation with PVCs_____

22. . Rate __50's BPM ___ Rhythm __irregular ___ P Wave _multiple saw toothed P waves ___PR Interval __not measurable ___ QRS Complex _narrow __ QT Interval __not measurable___ QTc __not measurable___ T Wave _ present but distorted by P waves_ Other __none __ Interpretation __atrial flutter with variable conduction block _____

23. . Rate __110 BPM ___ Rhythm __irregular ___ P Wave _multiple and undulating ___PR Interval __not measurable ___ QRS Complex _narrow __ QT Interval__0.36 seconds ___ QTc __0.445 seconds ___ T Wave _present with some distortions because of P waves _ Other __none__ Interpretation __atrial fibrillation with rapid ventricular response _____ (in order to calculate corrected QT interval, the method of averaging QTc1 and QTc2 was done. RR interval between sixth and seventh ventricular beat from the left was considered for QTc1 and the RR interval between seventh and eighth beat was taken for QTc2.

24. . Rate __63 BPM ___ Rhythm __regular ___ P Wave _present ___PR Interval __0.24 seconds ___ QRS Complex _narrow __ QT Interval__ 0.44 seconds ___ QTc __0.449 seconds ___ T Wave _present _ Other __pacer spikes __ Interpretation __atrial paced rhythm _____

25. . Rate __40's in irregular rhythms and 79 BPM during regular rhythm ___ Rhythm __irregular turns to regular ___ P Wave _multiple P waves in irregular rhythms and single preceding P wave during regular rhythm ___PR Interval __0.20 seconds in regular rhythm without any prolongation ___ QRS Complex _narrow except in one QRS complex __ QT Interval__ 0.36 seconds ___ QTc __not measured___ T Wave _missing during some complexes _ Other __none __ Interpretation __second-degree Type II (Mobitz type II) heart block with a PVC turning to regular sinus rhythm_____

26. . Rate __60 BPM ___ Rhythm __irregular ___ P Wave _absent or inverted ___PR Interval __ varying ___ QRS Complex _0.14 seconds __ QT Interval__ 0.54 seconds ___ QTc __ 0.54 seconds ___ T Wave _in the opposite direction of QRS complex _ Other __regular PVCs__ Interpretation __junctional rhythm with bundle branch block and bigeminal PVC _____

27. . Rate __80's BPM ___ Rhythm __irregular ___ P Wave _multiple and undulating ___PR Interval __not measurable ___ QRS Complex _narrow __ QT Interval__ 0.44 seconds ___ QTc __0.509 seconds ___ T Wave _present but sometimes distorted with P waves _ Other __one PVC__ Interpretation __atrial fibrillation with controlled ventricular response and PVC_____

28. . Rate __75 BPM ___ Rhythm __irregular at one point___ P Wave _present ___PR Interval __0.24 seconds ___ QRS Complex _narrow __ QT Interval__0.42 seconds ___ QTc __0.47 seconds ___ T Wave _present _ Other __one PAC __ Interpretation __sinus rhythm with first-degree heart block and one PAC (second beat from the right)_____

29. . Rate __90's BPM ___ Rhythm __irregular ___ P Wave _multiple ___PR Interval __not measurable ___ QRS Complex _narrow__ QT Interval__ 0.36 seconds ___ QTc __0.466 seconds ___ T Wave _present _ Other __none __ Interpretation __atrial fibrillation with a controlled ventricular response _____

30. . Rate __93 BPM ___ Rhythm __regular ___ P Wave _present ___PR Interval __0.12 seconds ___ QRS Complex _narrow __ QT Interval__ 0.32 seconds ___ QTc __ 0.413 seconds ___ T Wave _present _ Other __none __ Interpretation __normal sinus rhythm _____

31. . Rate __83 BPM ___ Rhythm __regular ___ P Wave _present ___PR Interval __0.20 seconds ___ QRS Complex _0.16 seconds __ QT Interval__0.44 seconds ___ QTc __0.519 seconds ___ T Wave _present _ Other __none __ Interpretation __sinus rhythm with bundle branch block _____

32. . Rate __ 115 BPM during tachycardia and 65 BPM during regular rhythm___ Rhythm __regular with variable rate ___ P Wave _present ___PR Interval __0.20 in regular rhythm ___ QRS Complex _narrow __ QT Interval__ 0.44 seconds in regular rhythm and not measurable in tachycardia ___ QTc __0.464 seconds in regular rhythm ___ T Wave _present _ Other __none__ Interpretation __paroxysmal supraventricular tachycardia (PS VT) turns to regular sinus rhythm _____

33. . Rate __71 BPM ___ Rhythm __regular ___ P Wave _present but inverted ___PR Interval __0.12 seconds ___ QRS Complex _narrow __ QT Interval__0.40 seconds ___ QTc __0.436 seconds ___ T Wave _present _ Other __none __ Interpretation __accelerated junctional rhythm _____

34. . Rate __30's BPM ___ Rhythm __irregular ___ P Wave _absent in one beat ___PR Interval __ 0.20 seconds___ QRS Complex _narrow __ QT Interval__0.44 seconds ___ QTc __ 0.367 seconds ___ T Wave _present _ Other __present of 2.68 seconds pause __ Interpretation __sinus bradycardia with 2.68 seconds pause and junctional beat_____

35. . Rate __88 BPM ___ Rhythm __regular with the one irregular beat ___ P Wave _present except in one beat ___PR Interval __0.18 seconds ___ QRS Complex _narrow (0.08 seconds)__ QT Interval__0.40 seconds ___ QTc __ 0.485 seconds ___ T Wave _present _ Other __pacer spike __ Interpretation __ventricular paced rhythm _____

36. . Rate __40's BPM ___ Rhythm __irregular ___ P Wave _multiple ___PR Interval __variable ___ QRS Complex _missing in some beats__ QT Interval__0.40 seconds ___ QTc __not

measured ____ T Wave _missing in some beats _ Other __none __ Interpretation __second-degree Type I (Mobitz type I) heart block _____

37. . Rate __68 BPM ____ Rhythm __regular ____ P Wave _present ____PR Interval __0.24 seconds ___ QRS Complex _narrow __ QT Interval__0.44 seconds ___ QTc __0.469 seconds ____ T Wave _present _ Other __none __ Interpretation __ sinus rhythm with first-degree heart block _____

38. . Rate __107 BPM ____ Rhythm __regular ____ P Wave _present but buried in T wave ___PR Interval __not measurable ___ QRS Complex _narrow __ QT Interval__ 0.44 seconds ___ QTc __ 0.588 seconds ____ T Wave _present _ Other __none __ Interpretation __sinus tachycardia _____

39. . Rate __30's BPM ____ Rhythm __irregular ____ P Wave _not seen ___PR Interval __not measurable ___ QRS Complex _narrow __ QT Interval__0.54 seconds ___ QTc __not measured___ T Wave _present _ Other __pacer spikes__ Interpretation __pacemaker failure to capture _____

40. . Rate __75 BPM ____ Rhythm __regular ____ P Wave _multiple saw toothed ___PR Interval __not measurable ___ QRS Complex _narrow __ QT Interval__ not measurable ___ QTc __not measurable___ T Wave _present but distorted by P waves _ Other __none __ Interpretation __ atrial flutter with a 3 :1 conduction block_____

41. . Rate __93 BPM during regular rhythm and 166 BPM during tachycardia ____ Rhythm __irregular ____ P Wave _present during regular rhythm and not seen during tachycardia ___PR Interval __0.18 seconds during regular rhythm ___ QRS Complex _narrow __ QT Interval__0.36 seconds during regular rhythm___ QTc __ 0.443 seconds in regular rhythm___ T Wave _present but distorted during tachycardia _ Other __one PAC (fifth beat from the left) __ Interpretation __sinus rhythm with PAC initiating supraventricular tachycardia _____

42. . Rate __50's BPM ____ Rhythm __irregular ____ P Wave _present ____PR Interval __varying ___ QRS Complex _ 0.12 seconds__ QT Interval__ 0.40 seconds ___ QTc __not measured ____ T Wave _present _ Other __missing QRS complex __ Interpretation __second-degree type I (Mobitz type I) heart block_____

43. . Rate __68 BPM ____ Rhythm __regular ____ P Wave _present ____PR Interval __0.20 seconds ___ QRS Complex _narrow __ QT Interval__ 0.36 seconds ___ QTc __ 0.384 seconds ____ T Wave _present _ Other __none __ Interpretation __normal sinus rhythm _____

44. . Rate __60's BPM ____ Rhythm __irregular___ P Wave _multiple and undulating ___PR Interval __not measurable ___ QRS Complex _narrow__ QT Interval__ 0.38 seconds ___ QTc __ 0.411 seconds ___ T Wave _present but distorted _ Other __none __ Interpretation __atrial fibrillation _____(even though some saw toothed P waves are seen, it is not considered as atrial flutter because in atrial flutter P waves are mostly of uniform shape).

45. . Rate __115 BPM ___ Rhythm __regular ___ P Wave _present ___PR Interval __0.14 seconds ___ QRS Complex _narrow __ QT Interval__ 0.34 seconds ___ QTc __0.463 seconds ____ T Wave _ present _ Other __none __ Interpretation __sinus tachycardia _____

46. . Rate __34 BPM during bradycardia and 107 BPM during tachycardia ___ Rhythm __irregu-lar ___ P Wave _inverted and missing in some beats ___PR Interval __not measurable ___ QRS Complex _narrow __ QT Interval__0.52 seconds ___ QTc __not measured___ T Wave _present _ Other __none __ Interpretation __junctional rhythm turns to tachycardia (possible tachy-brady syndrome)_____

47. . Rate __50's BPM ___ Rhythm __irregular ___ P Wave _saw toothed ___PR Interval __not measurable ___ QRS Complex _narrow __ QT Interval__ not measured___ QTc __not mea-sured___ T Wave _distorted by P waves _ Other __none __ Interpretation __atrial flutter with variable conduction block _____

48. Rate __50's BPM ___ Rhythm __irregular___ P Wave _present ___PR Interval __0.14 seconds ___ QRS Complex _narrow __ QT Interval__ 0.32 seconds ___ QTc __not measured___ T Wave _present_ Other __presence of early beats at regular interval__ Interpretation __sinus bradycar-dia with a bigeminal PAC _____

49. . Rate __75 BPM ___ Rhythm __regular ___ P Wave _present ___PR Interval __0.30 seconds ___ QRS Complex _wide (0.16 seconds) __ QT Interval__ 0.46 seconds ___ QTc __0.514 seconds ___ T Wave _present _ Other __pacer spikes __ Interpretation __atrial paced rhythm with bundle branch block_____

50. . Rate __regular rhythm at 79 BPM and tachycardia at 150 BPM___ Rhythm __irregular ___ P Wave _present except in tachycardia ___PR Interval __0.16 seconds during regular rhythm ___ QRS Complex _narrow during regular rhythm and wide in tachycardia __ QT Interval__ 0.42 seconds in regular rhythm ___ QTc __ 0.47 seconds in regular rhythm ___ T Wave _ present in regular rhythm_ Other __one early beat (fifth beat from the left) and presence of P wave prior to tachycardia __ Interpretation __ underlying sinus rhythm with a PAC having supraventricular tachycardia with aberrant conduction (not ventricular tachycardia because of the presence of ini-tiating P wave)_____

51. . Rate __80's BPM ___ Rhythm __irregular ___ P Wave _multiple and undulating ___PR Interval __not measurable ___ QRS Complex _narrow __ QT Interval__ not measured___ QTc __not measured___ T Wave _distorted by P waves _ Other __none __ Interpretation __atrial fibrillation with a controlled ventricular response_____

52. . Rate __ 136 BPM ___ Rhythm __regular ___ P Wave _present ___PR Interval __0.18 sec-onds ___ QRS Complex _narrow __ QT Interval__0.26 seconds ___ QTc __ 0.383 seconds ___ T Wave _present _ Other __none __ Interpretation __sinus tachycardia _____

53. . Rate __60 BPM ___ Rhythm __ regular___ P Wave _present ___PR Interval __0.16 seconds ___ QRS Complex _narrow __ QT Interval__ 0.40 seconds ___ QTc __ 0.404 seconds ___ T Wave _present _ Other __none __ Interpretation __normal sinus rhythm _____

54. . Rate __62 BPM in regular and 150 BPM in tachycardia___ Rhythm __irregular ___ P Wave _ present during regular rhythm ___PR Interval __0.12 seconds ___ QRS Complex _narrow in regular rhythm and wide during tachycardia __ QT Interval__ 0.38 seconds during regular rhythm___ QTc __0.384 seconds during regular rhythm ___ T Wave _present during regular rhythm_ Other __presence of fusion beats (4th beat during tachycardia)__ Interpretation __sinus rhythm with the short run of VT with a fusion beats in between _____

55. . Rate __30's BPM during bradycardia and 68 BPM during regular rhythm___ Rhythm __irregular ___ P Wave _multiple ___PR Interval __variable ___ QRS Complex _ narrow __ QT Interval__0.40 seconds ___ QTc __not measured___ T Wave _present_ Other __missing QRS complex __ Interpretation __second-degree Type I (Mobitz type I) heart block _____

56. . Rate __51 BPM ___ Rhythm __regular ___ P Wave _present ___PR Interval __0.20 seconds ___ QRS Complex _wide (0.20 seconds) __ QT Interval__0.52 seconds ___ QTc __ 0.487 seconds ___ T Wave _present_ Other __none __ Interpretation __sinus bradycardia with a bundle branch block _____

57. . Rate __80's BPM ___ Rhythm __irregular ___ P Wave _multiple and undulating ___PR Interval __not measurable ___ QRS Complex _narrow __ QT Interval__0.34 seconds ___ QTc __ 0.412 seconds ___ T Wave _present_ Other __none __ Interpretation __ atrial fibrillation with controlled ventricular response_____

58. . Rate __Paced rhythm at the 71 BPM and tachycardia at 125 BPM___ Rhythm __irregular___ P Wave _& except tachycardia ___PR Interval __constant ___ QRS Complex _narrow except tachycardia__ QT Interval __not measurable___ QTc __not measurable___ T Wave _seen except in tachycardia _ Other __pacer spikes__ Interpretation __ventricular pacing rhythm with short run of ventricular tachycardia _____

59. . Rate __60 BPM ___ Rhythm __regular ___ P Wave _present___ PR Interval __0.20 seconds ___ QRS Complex _0.12 seconds __ QT Interval__0.4 server seconds ___ QTc __ 0.4 seconds ___ T Wave _present_ Other __none __ Interpretation __sinus rhythm with bundle branch block____

60. . Rate __60's BPM ___ Rhythm __irregular ___ P Wave _multiple and undulating ___PR Interval __not measurable ___ QRS Complex _narrow __ QT Interval__0.40 seconds ___ QTc __ 0.431 seconds ___ T Wave _present with distortions from P wave _ Other __none__ Interpretation __atrial fibrillation with controlled ventricular response _____

12 Lead EKG Interpretation

Answer key

1. Rate and Rhythm __sinus rhythm at 75 BPM __ Axis __normal axis__ BBB/ Hemiblock __none __ Enlargement - Atria/ Ventricle ____ not seen ____ Ischemia/ Infarction __none __ Other ____ motion artifact in lead V2 and V3__ Interpretation __normal sinus rhythm at 75 beats per minute with some motion artifact ____

2. Rate and Rhythm __ sinus rhythm with a first degree AV block (PR-0.28 seconds) __ Axis __left axis deviation (negative lead aVF and positive lead I) __ BBB/ Hemiblock __ left bundle branch block (negative V1, positive lead I and V6 with a wide QRS complex) __Enlargement - Atria/ Ventricle____ left atrial enlargement (notched and wide P in lead III, aVF and V1) ____ Ischemia/ Infarction __ none __ Other ___none __ Interpretation __left bundle branch block with a first degree AV block and left axis deviation ____

3. Rate and Rhythm __ sinus rhythm at 68 BPM __ Axis __left axis deviation __ BBB/ Hemiblock __ left anterior fascicle block (left axis, qR pattern in lead I and aVL, qS pattern in inferior leads) __Enlargement - Atria/ Ventricle ____ left ventricular hypertrophy (R aVL+ S V3 = 36)____ Ischemia/ Infarction __ infero-lateral T wave inversion __ Other ___none __ Interpretation __sinus rhythm with left anterior fascicular block and LVH with Infero lateral ischemia ____

4. Rate and Rhythm __ atrial fibrillation at 60's BPM __ Axis __right axis deviation (negative lead I and positive aVF) __ BBB/ Hemiblock __ none __Enlargement - Atria/ Ventricle ____ none ____ Ischemia/ Infarction __ anterior infarct (presence of deep S waves in anterior leads) __ Other ____ none __ Interpretation __atrial fibrillation with right axis deviation and old anterior infarct ____

5. Rate and Rhythm __ sinus rhythm at 83 BPM __ Axis __normal axis __ BBB/ Hemiblock__ none __Enlargement - Atria/ Ventricle ____ none ____ Ischemia/ Infarction __ inferior ST segment elevation with possible old anterior infarct (prominent S waves in precordial leads)__ Other ___ST segment depression in V1 and V2 (mirror image of inferior infarction)__ Interpretation __inferior STEMI with the possible old antero-septal infarct ____

6. Rate and Rhythm__sinus rhythm at 75 BPM__ Axis __normal axis __ BBB/ Hemiblock__none __Enlargement - Atria/ Ventricle____none ____ Ischemia/ Infarction__up to 1 mm ST segment elevation in lateral leads __ Other ___none __ Interpretation __lateral STEMI ____

7. Rate and Rhythm __atrial pacing at 63 BPM __ Axis __normal axis __ BBB/ Hemiblock__none __Enlargement - Atria/ Ventricle___none ____ Ischemia/ Infarction __not seen__ Other ___none __ Interpretation __atrial paced rhythm (Note that the pacer spike is not visible in every leads and this should not make the interpreter think that pacemaker is not working. Since all the leads are capturing at the same time, if you see a pacer spike in one lead which means it is a pacer rhythm.)

8. Rate and Rhythm__atrial fibrillation at 90's BPM __ Axis __normal axis __ BBB/ Hemiblock__ none __Enlargement - Atria/ Ventricle___not seen ____ Ischemia/ Infarction__not seen __ Other

____saw toothed P waves in lead V1 (Crista Terminalis effect as mentioned in chapter 6)__ Interpretation __atrial fibrillation with a controlled ventricular response_____

9.Rate and Rhythm__atrial 100 BPM and ventricular 36 BPM __ Axis __normal axis __ BBB/ Hemiblock__none __Enlargement - Atria/ Ventricle___none ____ Ischemia/ Infarction__not seen __ Other ____atrioventricular dissociation __ Interpretation __third degree heart block ____

10. Rate and Rhythm__sinus rhythm with 65 BPM __ Axis __left axis deviation__ BBB/ Hemiblock__ none __Enlargement - Atria/ Ventricle___not seen ____ Ischemia/ Infarction__inferior Q waves and T wave inversion in lead III and aVF __ Other ___none __ Interpretation __sinus rhythm with possible old inferior infarct and possible inferior ischemia ____

11. Rate and Rhythm__ sinus rhythm at 79 BPM__ Axis __normal axis __ BBB/ Hemiblock__not seen __Enlargement - Atria/ Ventricle___none ____ Ischemia/ Infarction__isolated deep S wave in lead III __ Other ____ QTc 0.485 seconds __ Interpretation __sinus rhythm with the long QT interval ____

12. Rate and Rhythm__ sinus rhythm at 63 bpm __ Axis __normal axis __ BBB/ Hemiblock__none __Enlargement - Atria/ Ventricle___not seen ____ Ischemia/ Infarction__ up to 1 mm Q waves in lateral leads __ Other ___none __ Interpretation __sinus rhythm with possible old lateral infarct ____

13. Rate and Rhythm__sinus rhythm at 75 BPM__ Axis __normal axis __ BBB/ Hemiblock__none __Enlargement - Atria/ Ventricle___left ventricular hypertrophy with strain pattern (tall R waves with characteristic ST depression in precordial leads) ____ Ischemia/ Infarction__inferolateral T wave inversion (subendocardial ischemia from LVH)__ Other ____ none__ Interpretation __sinus rhythm with the left ventricular hypertrophy ____

14. Rate and Rhythm__sinus rhythm at 100 BPM__ Axis __left axis deviation __ BBB/ Hemiblock__right bundle branch block and left anterior fascicular block (bifascicular block) __Enlargement - Atria/ Ventricle___none ____ Ischemia/ Infarction__not seen __ Other ____ none __ Interpretation __sinus rhythm with bifascicular block ____

15. Rate and Rhythm__sinus rhythm at 68 BPM __ Axis __extreme right axis deviation __ BBB/ Hemiblock__ none __Enlargement - Atria/ Ventricle___not seen ____ Ischemia/ Infarction__anterior ST segment elevation in lead V2 in V3, old septal and anterolateral infarct (deep S waves) __ Other ___none __ Interpretation __sinus rhythm with the extreme right axis deviation and anterior STEMI with the old septal anterolateral infarct ____

16. Rate and Rhythm__sinus rhythm at 75 BPM __ Axis __left axis deviation __ BBB/ Hemiblock__ left anterior fascicular block __Enlargement - Atria/ Ventricle___left ventricular hypertrophy ____ Ischemia/ Infarction__anterior ST segment elevation __ Other ___none __ Interpretation __sinus rhythm with the left anterior fascicle block and anterior STEMI ____

17. Rate and Rhythm__sinus rhythm at the 75 BPM__ Axis __normal axis __ BBB/ Hemiblock__ left branch block __Enlargement - Atria/ Ventricle__left ventricular hypertrophy ____ Ischemia/ Infarction__not assessed__ Other ____ none __ Interpretation __sinus rhythm with left bundle branch block and left ventricular hypertrophy ____

18. Rate and Rhythm__sinus rhythm at 83 BPM __ Axis __normal axis __ BBB/ Hemiblock__none __Enlargement - Atria/ Ventricle___none ____ Ischemia/ Infarction__ inferior STEMI __ Other ___ none __ Interpretation __ sinus rhythm with the inferior STEMI ____

19. Rate and Rhythm__sinus rhythm at 68 BPM __ Axis __left axis deviation__ BBB/ Hemiblock__none __Enlargement - Atria/ Ventricle___ left ventricular hypertrophy ____ Ischemia/ Infarction__ old anterior infarct __ Other ___none __ Interpretation __sinus rhythm with left axis deviation and possible old anterior infarct ____

20. Rate and Rhythm__sinus rhythm at the 65 BPM __ Axis __normal axis __ BBB/ Hemiblock__ none__Enlargement - Atria/ Ventricle ____ none ____ Ischemia/ Infarction __ inferior Q waves__ Other ____ none __ Interpretation __normal sinus rhythm with the possible old inferior infarct ____

Appendix A

Summary of 12 lead EKG Interpretations			
Rate and Rhythm	• Six second method • Counting small box method • Presence of PQRST and its characteristics • Look for intervals		
Axis	look at lead **I** and **aVF** (*consider entire QRS complex for axis determination*)		
	Vertical axis (Consider Lead **I** and **aVF**)	Normal axis	Lead **I** and **aVF** positive
		Right axis	Lead **I** negative and **aVF** positive
		Left axis	Lead **I** positive and **aVF** negative
	Horizontal axis (Look at **V1**, **V2** and **V5**, **V6**)	Anterior axis	Positive **V1** and **V2**
		Posterior axis	Positive **V5** and **V6**
Bundle branch block	• Look at lead **I**, **V1** and **V6** (*only last half of the QRS complex*) • It require QRS duration > 0.12 sec		
	RBBB	Negative lead **I** and **V6** and positive **V1**	
	LBBB	Negative lead **V1** and positive lead **I** and **V6** (R or R')	
Hemiblock	look at lead **I** and **aVF**		
	Left anterior hemiblock (LAHB)	Left axis deviation	Lead **I** positive and **aVF** negative
		qR complex in the lateral limb leads	Lead **I** and **aVL**
		rS complex in the in inferior leads	Lead **II**, **III** and **aVF**
		Delayed intrinsicoid deflection (time for R wave peak)	In aVL >0.45 seconds
		Do not diagnose LAHB in presence of inferior infarct (prominent **Q** in lead **II**, **III** and **aVF**)	
	Left posterior hemiblock (LPHB)	Right axis deviation	lead **I** negative and **aVF** positive
		rS pattern in lead **I** and **aVL** tall R waves in **II**, **III** and **aVF**	This goes with right axis deviation
		Looks similar to S1Q3T3 pattern as in pulmonary embolism	
Chamber enlargement	Right atrial enlargement	Narrow and tall **P** wave in lead **II** and **V1**	P pulmonale
	Left atrial enlargement	Wide P wave with notching in lead **III**, **aVF** and **V1**	
	Right ventricular hypertrophy	Tall **R** waves in **V1**, **V2** and deep **S** waves in **V5** and **V6**	
		Right axis deviation	Negative lead **I** and positive **aVF**
	Left ventricular hypertrophy	Left axis deviation)	(Positive lead **I** and negative **aVF**
		Down sloping **ST** and inverted **T** wave in lateral leads	LV Strain pattern
		R in **aVL** plus S in **V3** > 28 mm in men and >20 mm in	Cornell criteria

Summary of 12 lead EKG Interpretations- Cont...

Ischemia	ST segment depression and T wave inversion	Lead I, aVL, V5 and V6	Lateral wall (Left circumflex artery)
		Lead II, III and aVF	Inferior leads (Right coronary artery)
		Lead V1, V2, V3 and V4	Anterior wall (LAD territory)
Infarction	Acute myocardial infarction	ST segment elevation in the target area with ST segment depression and T wave inversion in the opposite area	Reciprocal changes
	Old myocardial infarction	Presence of large Q waves in target areas	At least > 1 mV
Other abnormalities	Pulmonary embolism	Prominent S in lead I, Q wave and inverted T wave in lead III	S1Q3T3 pattern
		Right ventricular strain pattern	ST depression in V1-V3
		Sinus tachycardia	
		New incomplete RBBB	
	Hyperkalemia (depending on serum level)	Tall peaked T waves	
		ST segment depression	
		Various bundle branch block	
		Severe bradycardia with AV block	
		V tach/V-Fib	
	Pericarditis	PR segment depression	
		Generalized ST segment elevation	
	Hypocalcaemia	prolonged QTc	
		Flat or inverted T waves	
		Prolonged ST segment without increase in T wave duration	
	Hypercalcemia	Short QTc	
		PR segment prolongation	
	Hypomagnesaemia	Peak T wave	
		Prominent T wave	
		prolonged QRS	
		ST segment depression	
		Polymorphic ventricular tachycardia	
	Pericardial effusion or Cardiac tamponade	Low voltage EKG	
		Electrical alternance	Beat to beat change in amplitude

Index

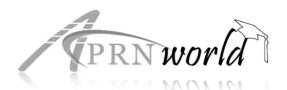

About us

APRN WORLD is an innovative publishing and training company focusing on delivering quality education and training, that is *affordable*, *accessible* and *meaningful* for students and working professionals.

How we **differ?**

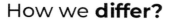

- Powered by *m learning*
- Highly refined training methodology
- In depth result analysis and feedback
- Seamless integration across devise platforms
- Unparalleled academic and technical support

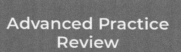

Advanced Practice Review

AG-ACNP
AGNP
FNP
PMHNP

Critical Care Review

CCRN
CMC
CSC
PCCN

Pre-Licensure Review

NCLEX RN

CE Courses

Advanced Arrhythmia
and many more

on sale

Basic Concepts of EKG, Cardiac Pharmacology, EKG pocket card, Advanced Arrhythmia DVD, Certification Exam Review courses
and many more

GET IN TOUCH WITH US

 3200 Guasti Road, Suite 100, City of Ontario, California, 91761

 9099074144   support@aprnworld.com   www.aprnworld.com

Made in the USA
Middletown, DE
25 January 2021